Surprise Child

Finding Hope in Unexpected Pregnancy

LESLIE LEYLAND FIELDS

SURPRISE CHILD

Trade Paperback ISBN 978-1-4000-7094-7
eBook ISBN 978-0-307-49994-3

Published in the United States by WaterBrook, an imprint of the Crown Publishing Group, a division of Penguin Random House LLC, New York.

WATERBROOK® and its deer colophon are registered trademarks of Penguin Random House LLC.

Library of Congress Cataloging-in-Publication Data
Fields, Leslie Leyland, 1957-
    Surprise child : finding hope in unexpected pregnancy / Leslie Leyland Fields. — 1st ed.
        p. cm.
    Includes bibliographical references.
    ISBN 1-4000-7094-5
    1. Pregnant women—Religious life. 2. Pregnancy—Religious aspects—Christianity. 3. Pregnancy, Unwanted—Religious aspects—Christianity. I. Title.
    BV4529.18.F54 2006
    248.8'431—dc22

                                                    2005023121

Printed in the United States of America
2017

10 9 8 7 6 5 4

Praise for
Surprise Child

"Many women today find an unexpected pregnancy too much to bear… If only they could read *Surprise Child* to know they are not alone, they are not freaks, they are not unworthy. *Surprise Child* brings 'realness' to the issue that not all pregnancies are planned by us but are always planned by God."

—YVETTE MAHER, vice president of Community
Impact Outreach, Focus on the Family

"Leslie Fields has at last dealt with an issue that deeply affects all of us regardless of race, culture, or economic status. Sharing from her own personal experience as well as utilizing the experiences of others, Fields compassionately addresses the deepest feelings and concerns of those facing an 'unplanned' pregnancy. *Surprise Child* should be required reading for anyone who works or serves in a related counseling field or ministry and would be a tremendous benefit to current or future mothers and families everywhere."

—RAUL REYES, president and executive director
of Life Network

"After twenty-one years of marriage and two teenagers nearly grown and gone, the last thing my husband and I expected was a 'surprise child.' I wish I'd had this book as a companion. Leslie Leyland Fields offers a practical yet poignant look at the wrestling, the emotionally tumultuous joy that characterizes an unexpected pregnancy. She points us to the hope that while this child may have been unplanned by us, he or she was not unplanned by God."

—JOANNA WEAVER, author of *Having a Mary Heart in a Martha World*

"I felt terribly alone when I faced my crisis pregnancy. I wish I had been able to read this book then to discover how many other women were facing this trauma—and overcoming! Leslie Fields makes it clear that, despite how overpowering our emotions make it seem, we are not alone, and we are not trapped."

—HEATHER GEMMEN, international speaker and best-selling author of *Startling Beauty: My Journey from Rape to Restoration*

Surprise Child

To Duncan, my life partner,
who labored with me, sharing the unspeakable
wonder and hurt of birth
six times over.

And to the Creator
who fashions every child
in the very image
and beauty
of God's own self.

Contents

Contents

Four years ago I walked into the bathroom, hand clenched around a white cellophane-wrapped stick. Three minutes later the bathroom door opened, and my face was white. In a tiny centimetered window no bigger than my fingernail a faint line slowly emerged, then solidified. It was the face of another human being—one I had not asked for. Surely my life was over.

Less than two years later it would happen again. In spite of—everything: our fastidious use of birth control, our ages, our frantically stressful lives, our full household. In spite of all this, the line appeared again and with it a maelstrom of emotions: anger, denial, incredulity, grief—all familiar visitors from the first surprise pregnancy. But this time all descended with an intensity that nearly crushed me.

God had personally delivered to my door my second worst fear. My greatest fear was that I would lose my husband or one of my four children. My second fear, however irrational, was that God would give me another child—that after loving and lavishing and persevering through the infancies and toddlerhoods of three highly energetic boys and one iron-willed daughter, and while still pouring out my best energy and resources to these beloved human beings, he would make me start again, at the very beginning. Just as I had emerged into relative light and safety. Now another. Do it again. And then another. And not pregnancies only. Yes, the weight gain, nausea, stretch marks, sleepless nights, varicose veins, but far more, the all-night feedings, leaking breasts, fevered weeks of teething, endless laundry, perpetual exhaustion, potty training... I knew it all intimately.

And so I cried, I protested, I prayed, alternating between anger and numbness, submission and rebellion. Must I give up my career? How will I do this? How do I make it through all those interminable nights? How do we fit six kids in this house? How do we send them all to college? What will I say to the shocked faces in the grocery store? How do I find joy in this?

In the midst of the quaking of my world, there were two things I knew for certain. God is the maker of life. And somehow I must find a way to receive with open hands these children he had made. I had no choice but to choose this. This tiny creature would come, slipping from between my legs in that final gush into the doctor's hands and then mine, and how would I greet this precious first-seen face who already knew my voice, my smell, who knew me from the inside out? Would I cradle and behold him with joy, or would I contain his little body in my hands with resentment, apathy, bitterness? I must choose joy. But how would I get there? Who could help me travel this very long distance between my mourning and sobbing now and this necessary joy later?

Throughout both pregnancies I felt terribly alone. I did not belong to any identifiable group. Despite my expanding profile, I felt cut off from other pregnant women who glowed with expectation and delight; cut off from my peers at the college where I taught, who were openly puzzled about this derailment of my teaching career; cut off from women in my church and larger faith community who thrived on homeschooling and rejoiced over their every pregnancy, no matter how many children they had. When I finally ventured forth the news at church, my pastor greeted my somber announcement with a congratulatory pounding on my back and a crow of delight. I looked at him, dumbstruck. Didn't he understand that the coming of this new life was also a kind of death? Didn't he know how much I had given already and that I had no more left to give?

In my hunger and need, I began to look for books about unexpected pregnancy. The bookstore shelves were lined with either chirpy pregnancy journals and manuals that assumed a glad giddiness toward pregnancy or a host of birth-and-tell-all books written by highly educated women who had one or two children and who reveled in their own angst and ambivalence as mothers. I couldn't stomach either one. I also found a book, *Bitter Fruit: Women's Experiences of Unplanned Pregnancy, Abortion, and Adoption,* that presented the stories of women who had aborted their babies out of fear or discomfort or an unwillingness to alter their lifestyles. Those who elected to keep their child were bitter, resenting the child's needs and intrusion into their lives. I knew there was nothing here for me. *Am I really this alone?* I wondered.

Then I discovered a book that began to answer this question. *The Best Intentions* is a report compiled by the National Institutes of Health after a year of intensive focus on unexpected pregnancies. They report that 60 percent of all pregnancies in the United States are unplanned. That translates into three million women a year. Three million women find themselves pregnant at the wrong time in their lives: women who are single, middle-aged, with a houseful already, unemployed, at the top of their profession, just starting out…and everywhere in between. Three million women a year whose lives are radically interrupted. Half of those three million women choose to end the pregnancy.[1]

Where were these women? I began looking for them in the safest place I knew—online. Almost immediately they appeared: chat rooms and Web sites abounded, all of them a frenzy of impassioned dialogue. What I read in those places shocked and saddened me. I found my own desperation magnified across a hundred, a thousand lives. I found words and voices of women in every possible state of function and dysfunction, all of them facing an unexpected pregnancy and all of them feeling alone, desperate for help and answers.

I read the words of Jennifer,* who wrote:

> I am twenty-six and have a five-year-old.... She has recently started school and I am returning to college.... Her dad and I have been together ten years.... I was happy when my daughter started school as it meant I could finally follow my dreams.... Yesterday I found out I was pregnant.... I am scared to tell my partner, as I know he will be happy, as he wants more kids. I so don't want another baby in my life right now. Abortion was the first thing that crossed my mind, but I feel so selfish for even thinking that. We could provide a home for a baby, but I do not want the responsibility.... I am upset and have nowhere to turn.... Can anyone help?[2]

Suzanne, a teenager, wrote this:

> I am fifteen years old...and there is a very big chance I am pregnant.... I have talked to my boyfriend

---

* Throughout this book the use of only first names indicates the name has been changed to protect privacy. All quotes from individuals are from the author's personal interviews unless otherwise noted.

about what to do if I am pregnant and he just wants
me to get an abortion. He says he loves me but we
aren't ready for a baby.... If I told my mom I was
pregnant she would be so disappointed in me. She
would tell me I have to get an abortion.... I won't
get an abortion no matter what. And I also don't
want adoption.... I just need someone to talk to that
can help and give me some advice.[3]

Another woman, Lila, described her situation:

I just found out...I am pregnant and I do not see
how. I have never missed one pill. I am devastated.
I have four boys. My youngest is seven months old.
I love my boys so much, but we can't afford another
one and I have always been against abortion. But I
do not know what else to do. My husband wants me
to have it done. Actually he is putting a lot of pressure on me. But I do not think he gets how this is
affecting me. We made an appointment for this Friday to have it done and I am already beside myself.
Please, if anyone is out there, please help me.[4]

I was astounded that my personal crisis fit into a pattern
and context so huge and yet so concealed. I felt as though I
had uncovered a vast cave of silence, hidden from the world

of light and noise and everyday lives. It had been here all along, of course—and now I too had slipped into this subterranean space. But once I landed and saw how many others were there, I understood why the cries from that place were scarcely heard above. It was so intensely private from the very start: the making of love between a man and a woman, the family planning behind bedroom doors, the silent burrowing of sperm into egg, the secrets of the uterus. And once that child exists in the womb or at the family table, who will call her child unplanned, unexpected— implying failure, mistake, accident? Who will taint flesh of very flesh with this stigma? Yet what rescues this whole enterprise—what saves the pages of this book and the lives of the women and children who appear in it—is the possibility, no, the *probability* that transformation will take place.

Even before that transformation, I realized that my own isolation would not go away until I spoke the truth to those around me. It was not courage on my part; it was need—my distaste for dissembling, my inability to pretend that all was well all the time. As I met friends and acquaintances in the grocery-store aisles, my usual professional clothes replaced by leggings and maternity tops, my belly now well extended, I would explain carefully to questioning faces, "God has brought us a surprise." On good days I would smile, act as though this was all in hand, but if I knew the friend well, I did not try to smile. That is how I found out that some of those three million women were living right here in my own small town. My openness encouraged honesty in others, and through those months of pregnancy, through whispered conversations, I heard from so many:

"Yes, this happened to me. My last child was a complete shock!"

"I think I'm pregnant, Leslie—and I'm a grandmother! What shall I do?"

"I missed my period—I've got two other children. I can't handle another child!"

"I had an unplanned pregnancy a few years ago. I felt so alone. No one understood what I was going through."

"I knew having another child meant less time with my two girls. I didn't want to give that up."

"Mom, a girl in my class is going to have a baby—she's fourteen."

It seemed nearly every woman I knew had either experienced an unexpected pregnancy or was close to someone who had.

The statistics were gone. In their place were the solemn faces, voices, and expressions of women all around me, and nearly every story or conversation ended with a question or a cry for help. Though many were in situations more dire than mine, they still needed what I needed—not a sermon, not an elder's glib congratulations, not a pat on the back that everything will be fine, but another woman who is herself pregnant to walk beside them, someone else ahead of them who has birthed her surprise child, motioning toward hope and joy.

I have written this book from both places. Looking for solace, I began interviewing others and writing while I was in the midst of my pregnancies, still struggling, still facing the dark of the tunnel ahead. The quotes and stories throughout the book are derived from those interviews, except for a few taken from online message boards, which will be noted. I knew what to ask in the interview sessions, because I was asking for myself as well. Through this process I have come to know women in many life circumstances: Jill, unmarried, in her first year of teaching, wakes up one morning and discovers she is pregnant—and her boyfriend wants no part of it. Linda becomes pregnant after she is raped, and she gives her baby to an adoption agency. Trisha spent the last seventeen years of her life raising her four children, running a day care in her home. Her oldest is about to graduate; her youngest has just started school. Now she is free to enroll in college classes to begin her education and a career, but no, she is pregnant again. Teresa and her new husband are getting ready to retire and move to a warmer climate—and the pregnancy test reads positive. Bianca, a multitalented freshman in a musical theater program at an exclusive college, gets pregnant and must leave the program. Pam has had four miscarriages in a row and has decided she doesn't want another pregnancy—she cannot bear another miscarriage. And then she *is* pregnant again. Marianne is only sixteen when she misses her period. Her boyfriend is an alcoholic and doesn't want the baby. Each one here had her life interrupted, each one here has a child who came to her unbidden, and each one now cannot imagine her life without that child.

And I am among them. I am not the same woman who started this book. I began my pregnancies and this project in the darkness of anxiety, resistance, and fear. Five years later I stand outside in light and clean air, my two surprise children, Abraham and Micah, in my arms. I will share with you, month by month, chapter by chapter, the unfolding of these unexpected pregnancies just as they happened so that you will find yourself here somewhere along the way. During the weeks and months of pregnancy, fears can grow as rapidly and as tangibly as the fetus himself. I will voice these fears common to so many of us and will tell as honestly as possible what has come of them in others' lives and in my own.

All of us know that, essentially, we have three choices

before us. I do not pretend to be neutral—I will choose life every time. But some women may come to this book undecided about the life within them. Others may be deciding whether they will raise their surprise child themselves or will entrust their child to others. Others have decided to keep this baby, but the road ahead feels long and hard. My life circumstances allowed me to keep these two surprise children born to me. Not everyone can or should make the decision I did. But this book is written for every one of us. There are women here who have not chosen life and who speak honestly about that experience. Two other women tell deeply personal stories of giving their newborns to another family. In these pages we can gaze directly into other women's journeys through pregnancy and birth—women like you, who struggle with the reality of a coming child. Month by month, page by page, you may discover what is possible for your own life and the life of your child.

For the millions of women who will wake up one day to find themselves pregnant at the wrong time, at a hard time, at a difficult place in their lives—this book is for you. May you find the honesty, hope, and joy that I have found through these women's stories. And may you be given the strength to carry on.

The First Trimester

One

The Test

You have ovulated and an egg is traveling along one of the
fallopian tubes toward your uterus. During intercourse
one of the millions of sperm your partner has ejaculated
has fertilized the egg while still in the fallopian tube.
Your baby is a cluster of cells which multiply rapidly
as they continue the journey along the fallopian tube.
It arrives in your uterus and embeds itself in the uterine
lining. The placenta is beginning to form around it.
—*THE COMPLETE BOOK OF PREGNANCY
AND CHILDBIRTH*

As you do not know the path of the wind,
or how the body is formed in a mother's womb,
so you cannot understand the work of God,
the Maker of all things.
—ECCLESIASTES 11:5

How does it begin? The glances at the calendar, the waiting, though you do not even know you are waiting. And the checking every time you go to the bathroom. You know you're not and it can't be, and any day now…but it is days now, and now you know you are waiting, and it's hard to sleep at night, and it's hard to keep going with the other kids and work, so you go to the store.

At the store you check the aisles furtively, hoping you will not see anyone you know. There they are, the small boxes in neat rows just under the condoms, whose packaging promises beach romps and unearthly sexual delights. The irony does not escape you, but you cannot smile. Standing in line, you try to hide the box under your arm, wishing it were sanitary pads or douche or personal lubricant, anything else from the Aisle of Embarrassment than the product you are holding. Remember your face—let go, erase its tautness. What will you say if you see a friend? Say nothing, act oblivious, smile. No one needs to know.

The purchase comes home, the plastic bag holding an almost weightless package, yet the slim box so full of significance, so freighted with the possibility of upheaval, so…yes, the contents of this bag so *pregnant* with meaning. What other word?

I've done this many times before, bought so many different brands that I must read the directions each time. What is it with this one? How many days do I wait after a missed period? Morning urine or anytime? Pee in a cup or on a stick? Rinse under running water for how long or no rinse at all? Wait one minute or three or five? A pink line, a blue line, a double line, or any line at all?

This one is a stick wrapped in white cellophane, like a tampon, except I suddenly realize it is the opposite of a tampon—this is what you use when the bleeding doesn't start. I read the directions carefully. This matters so much my hands shake. I am making or unmaking someone's life, it feels. A chemistry experiment I am conducting in my own bathroom with the door locked tight. Who knew life and death could come in a kit like this from the drugstore? I pee on the white wand for the prescribed number of seconds, then set the wand on the counter by the sink. I have only three minutes to wait, and the announcement will come in the space of a window no bigger than my fingernail. I cannot stand before it; it is like looking into the face of God. I leave the bathroom to wait and catch a glimpse of my face in the mirror as I turn away: I am white, erased of hope and desire, empty, every part of my life suspended in that space…

In the bedroom the white walls. Out the window the ocean furrowing, spruce wavering, wind roughing every surface. I know I am taking this test just to hush the barking dogs of worry. How foolish to have wasted money on it. It is asking just one simple question: am I _____? I can't say the word. It's an ugly word, an intensely private, harsh-sounding two-syllable construction—the first syllable open on the vowel *e,* then ending on that hard *g,* and the second syllable a drop of the voice into a mumble. The word as bulky as the figures it describes. I know what it means, how it parses, the etymology: Latin, *pre* meaning "before," and *gnosci* meaning "birth." This knowledge brings me nothing, no comfort, no help.

And surely I am not. The four days waiting for blood are just stress. I'm teaching an extra class—fifteen extra hours in the classroom this week. Of course my body will register that! Five classes, so many students calling, needing me. My own children clinging, one son sick. Duncan gone all last week... Food, sleep—no time for these. Who can have a period under these conditions? No, hold on to that blood, no matter where it keeps. You need every drop of oxygen-carrying plasma to keep you upright. Smart body, this one of mine!

I found out later that they all did it too, the women I talked to. They all had reasons for knowing they were not, could not be! Devie was twenty and planning her wedding when, with hands shaking, she took the pregnancy test into her grandmother's bathroom. Trisha Pruitt was running around the track, coaching the junior-high track team, when it suddenly occurred to her that her period was late. *I've just been training hard,* she thought. *This happens whenever I'm running a lot of miles.* She didn't want to spend money on a home test. Her sister, a week later, finally bought one and brought it to her house and insisted she take it. Ella had just come back from a trip to South Africa and got very sick with the flu. Except she didn't get better, and her period still hadn't come. *I can't be pregnant. I have only one ovary, and all these years we haven't conceived. It's just the travel.* Randi missed her period but was so busy she didn't give it another thought. She was teaching full time and had just started her master's program. How wonderful that she didn't have to deal with the usual cramps and fatigue with her hectic schedule. Besides, *I only slept with him once, and it wasn't the right time of the month to get pregnant.* Teresa Carlson was in her early forties, she and her new husband thinking about retirement. She began not feeling well, spotting instead of her usual period. She knew something was wrong but didn't know what it was. *I can't be pregnant. I haven't been pregnant for fourteen years.* Michael Schwarz was dealing with postpartum blues with her five-month-old baby and a demanding three-year-old. She felt sick for several weeks but knew she couldn't be pregnant. *I'm nursing day and night. I just had a baby. It can't be!*

While each of us, alone, recites all the reasons we must not be, cannot be, the second hand ticks around its circuit, and it is time. The decision is rendered. Innocent or guilty? The death of parts of the life you know or the same life? Walk through the bathroom doorway, eyes locked on the white wand. The tiny window opens…

Yes, of course, there is a line. Else there is no story, no giving up, no reconciliation, nothing to say about the ferocity of a slowly gathering love. The cliché is suddenly, powerfully true: this is the first day of the rest of your life—and someone else's life as well.

And this life and your new life begin with a flood of raw emotions, most of them colored dark by fear, by all you think you cannot do, by all you do not yet know.

What did I do in those first minutes? I stood over the test stick frozen, my breath gone for seconds. Then suddenly with a convulsive shake I sucked in the air I had lost; my heart went mad with drumming; my hands fisted, then went limp. And then I began to run, shouting, looking for someone to help me carry this.

Some minutes later Duncan and I sat on the couch, staring at the walls, both silently spinning our own sticky webs. Then it hit me: twenty minutes into knowing that I was a new mother again, I was already a bad mother. I was already guilty. Something in me told me I was supposed to be happy. I remembered when trying to start our family, how I

longed for any line at all to say, "Yes, you are with child."
And the ecstasy of seeing that line for the first time!

I thought of a few women I knew with large families
who glow beatifically when they discover they are pregnant
again. Vicky, who simply shrugged and said, smiling, "Well,
I am kind of busy, but each one is from God—praise him!"
Why couldn't I be like her? And what of all the women I
knew and the millions I didn't know who would give up
anything they possessed for a child, even a child not their
own? How was it that I was given so easily what others long
for so desperately? I should have been grateful.

But I could find no gratitude within me, only the
knowledge of all that this meant. I knew how that single
blue line would grow, multiply, divide, and finally crown,
my body convulsing. Then the slip of the shoulders and the
birth of astonishment—such perfection! Someone utterly
new, never before known, never seen, breathing first gulps of
air, then sprawled on my chest, knowing me by the timbre
of my voice, my smell, and rooting toward my nipple—all
this would happen. This child would claim oxygen, my milk,
would cry for me alone, would sob through dark nights for
only me.

But what would I have to give him? I was exhausted just
remembering the requirements for a baby's life. Would I be
so depleted or sad or numb that I felt nothing, that I had no
room within me for the crazy dance of wonder to spin and

reel? Would I not have a blessing for this one as I'd had for the others? I felt like Isaac, the ancient patriarch of Israel, who was tricked into speaking all his inheritance and blessing to the wrong son. When the rightful heir, the other son, came to receive the blessing, it was too late. Isaac howled with the deceit and with his own emptiness—the blessing had been spoken away, and he had little left for his other son. *I must have a blessing left. Surely one more. But where will it come from? How will I get it?*

What did others do in that moment of knowing and then those first moments afterward?

When Trisha Pruitt looked at the line on the stick, she didn't trust it. She had gotten false readings from those tests before. But her sister insisted the tests were accurate. Trisha shook her head, knowing it wasn't true. Three days later, still no period. Her sister brought another test to her house and insisted she take it. Positive again. But she didn't feel pregnant, and she had always known before when she was. This time she and her husband, Steve, went together to the doctor to put an end to this. The doctor returned to the room smiling. "You're pregnant!" Steve and Trisha laughed in disbelief, then left the office as quickly as they could, each one silent. Their oldest son was graduating from high school that spring. They had been raising their four children for seventeen years already.

Michael Schwarz took the test and saw a faint line forming. It couldn't be… No, it was too faint, and besides, she was nursing nonstop. She hadn't had a period since the baby was born five months ago. She wrapped the test in toilet paper, hands shaking, and ran over to her friend's house next door. "What does this mean?" she asked anxiously, thrusting the stick in Candy's face. She took one look and pronounced, "Congratulations!" Michael burst into tears.

Ella, in the bathroom with the test, started out angry. Angry that she had to shell out eleven dollars just to find out she wasn't pregnant. She and her husband had tried for years for a third child and had given up, relieved, five years ago. They were happy just as they were. When the line showed up, she stared in disbelief. Though she was forty-three, she instantly felt like a teenage girl: caught, guilty. The messages she had been teaching her daughters played back in her head: *You have sex, you get pregnant! What do you expect?* She felt herself falling off a high cliff, falling into a black hole— angry, frustrated, despairing. All that must be given up. All that must be done over again.

All the reasons to resist, to protest, to believe you cannot do what is now being asked of you:

"I just got my last daughter into school."

"I was just about to find a job and be a grownup again."

"My boyfriend doesn't want the baby. What am I going to do?"

"My last pregnancy was so hard—and he was born early. We had so many troubles with him. I can't think of going through all that again."

"What about my job? Will I have to give up this career that I love?"

"Maternity clothes again? I'll strangle myself with leggings if I have to wear those again. And those billowing tops that make you like you're going to sail away in the first wind. Please—not those terrible clothes!"

"I never planned to have a child past forty. I feel too old."

"I know this sounds silly, but it's so depressing to me to think of gaining all that weight again. It takes so long to get rid of it. I finally like how I look. And now I have to wave that body I like good-bye."

"How old will I be when this one graduates—105 or something?"

"How will I bear the comments? the snide glances?
the gossip—'They breed like rabbits! Can you
believe she's having *another*?' "

"How will I tell my mother? She'll kill me!"

Linda Ross was stunned when she realized she was pregnant. She knew how it happened—how could she forget?
She was twenty, a virgin, dating an older man that summer
while on break, though she knew he wasn't right for her. She
had finished two years of Bible school, where she was training for some form of ministry. She was the first in her large
family to pursue higher education. Everyone was proud of
her. That night as she and her date drove to Linda's apartment, he took another road and ended up at the lake. It was
late, dark, no one around. And there he raped her, his more-
than-six-foot-tall body easily overcoming her five-foot frame.
Linda did not report the crime. She couldn't face the police;
she didn't want to shame her family. Though distraught, she
kept silent, wondering if she could return to school in the
fall. And then her period didn't come. Wasn't it bad enough
to be raped but then to conceive a child? She told no one,
packed her belongings, and flew to California, her mind and
spirit devastated.

It is hard for me to imagine the depth of Linda's trauma,
a conception born of force. In some circumstances, like hers,

knowing brings devastation and desperation. But in many other circumstances, something else is possible. The test can bring the beginning of peace. Carol Nelson wished she had taken the test sooner. She had four boys, two of them grown, and a baby, now thirteen months old. With each one she had known when she was pregnant, and she knew now that another one was coming. But how could she tell her husband? How could they afford yet another baby? How could she love another child? As the days and weeks went by, she grew increasingly worried, increasingly frantic, increasingly fearful. After six weeks she could stand it no longer and drove to the Crisis Pregnancy Center. She took the test; the director sat with her while the line took shape. Carol looked at the line, nodded, almost with relief, and within moments the two prayed together, bending their heads, the test stick resting between them. In those minutes, for the first time Carol began to feel a sense of peace. Someone else knew now—she was no longer alone. And now she had taken it to God himself.

Even in the midst of the voices of fear, there is already something to hold on to. The test reads positive, and you know. And knowing frees you from the greatest fear: what *if* I am pregnant? Though that one fear gives rise to a hundred, each one of us in these pages could at this point, even while questioning and grieving, begin moving again.

We are the first generation to have this immediate

answer to our paralyzing question. How did women go so long not knowing? No test and knowledge sudden as a hammer: the news delivered in one strike. Yes. No. Carry on then. Cry or laugh, weep, throw up your arms, leap, kneel—whatever must be done and felt begins that moment, that very second. The gun fires, and bang, you run. At least you move; at least you know. As hard as the knowing is, that it comes early and quickly is a great mercy. Because there is much work to be done.

And remember now an even greater mercy. You are trying to live out the next two or three years of your life in these thirty minutes, in one day. Everything you fear visits you in one crushing blow. You feel weak, vulnerable. You think you cannot do it. You are right—it is impossible to live it all, to answer all these deep needs and fears in a single hour or a single day or week. As each day passes, some of your fears will fade; some will disappear entirely; some may slowly become reality. But in this moment, you do not need to answer all the questions. There will be time in each day to find answers, to find reasons to hope.

Two

Telling

By the end of the second month, the embryo is
more human looking, about 1¹/₄ inches long from head
to buttocks…and weighs about ¹/₃ of an ounce.
It has a beating heart, and arms and legs
with the beginning of fingers and toes.
Bone starts to replace cartilage.
—*WHAT TO EXPECT WHEN YOU'RE EXPECTING*

My frame was not hidden from you
when I was made in the secret place.
When I was woven together
in the depths of the earth…
—PSALM 139:15

Now that you know for certain, whom will you tell? Maybe in the heat of the test-stick discovery, you ran screaming, blurting the news out to anyone who would listen. Or maybe you plunked that stick down in front of your husband, angry and disbelieving. For most women in committed relationships, this is not a step they have to think about—their partners are the first to know. The immediate load of knowing you are pregnant is so hard to carry alone that you are desperate to share it. Now. The telling itself begins a long journey that at least can be shared with the other.

This is my experience. Duncan and I had been married twenty-two years when Abraham was conceived, twenty-four with Micah. Our lives and selves had merged in almost every area. When the test stick colored, and when I cried out the news to him, we knew, without asking, that we would birth and raise these babies together just as we had made them. That was all we knew, but it was all that was needed at first.

This does not happen for everyone. Maybe you haven't

told yet because you know your partner will not want the baby. Or maybe he will and you do not. Maybe you don't even know if you will see him again. Or if you are a teenager, maybe this is more about your parents. How will you tell them? They'll be so angry. And no matter what you want to do, they may push you to get an abortion, or they'll want you to have the baby adopted. And what about your boyfriend? What if he rejects you and leaves? You agonize over these possibilities. You know others have lived them out.

Marianne was sixteen, a sophomore in high school, when she suspected she was pregnant. Home pregnancy tests weren't easily available then, but the signs were all there. After two months, when she was certain she was indeed pregnant, she told her boyfriend, who was eighteen. His response: *No baby. Get an abortion.* Marianne refused. She didn't have a plan yet. She had hoped to be a mother someday. Not this soon, but she could not end her baby's life. She was certain of that. Certain, too, that she couldn't tell her parents. Her mother in particular had such hopes for Marianne. She would be crushed, even furious. The weeks went by. Marianne went to school, came home, went about her life as she was supposed to, but inside she felt sick, exhausted, and lonely. Her boyfriend had betrayed her; she had betrayed her parents.

Eventually Marianne could hide it no longer. When her mother discovered that her youngest daughter was pregnant, her response was just as Marianne had anticipated: she was angry and hysterical. Determined that this baby would not ruin her daughter's life, she demanded an abortion. In spite of Marianne's vehement protests, her mother drove her to the clinic, and the abortion was done.

The next week was a nightmare. Marianne lost her faith in God, her faith in her parents, her hope of someday being a mother.

But this is not the end. The abortion procedure was not successful. Marianne, telling her story to me more than twenty years later, says, "I think God brought her back to me. I knew this child was going to be Laurel, my daughter. I cannot even explain to you what I felt when I found out the baby was still there. And once my parents knew I *was* going to have this baby, everything changed. My father came to me—he was crying—and said, 'We're going to keep this baby. Don't worry. You can stay here with us. Everything is going to be okay.' "

Marianne went on to raise her daughter herself. Later that spring, after our interview, she was flying to see Laurel graduate from college with top honors.

Dana had just started college. Since she was the daughter of a military officer, her unexpected pregnancy at age twenty with an enlisted soldier was never made public. Her father suggested she travel with him to Mexico for an abortion, to bring a quick end to a problem he did not want to face. If she refused the abortion, he threatened to cut her and the baby off entirely. She would have to leave home, and she would have no further financial support from her parents, no money for college.

Dana refused to go. Though she had never envisioned herself with a baby at twenty, she could not get rid of it. She moved to another state, to a town where she had lived while in high school. She got two jobs, working in a cannery and as a nanny, and shared a small house with roommates. One morning, at seven and a half months along, Dana felt weak and sick. She went home from work early, and only a few hours later her daughter was born in the military base hospital. The baby was tiny, just under four pounds, with beautiful black hair. For a few short moments, Dana held her with unspeakable astonishment, until a nurse came and whisked the newborn away "to clean her up."

Dana never saw her baby again. Since she was a dependent in a military hospital, all decisions had to go through her father. The hospital notified him when Dana checked in and then informed him of the birth. His response was immediate and clear: the baby was to be given to an adoption agency. The doctor then issued orders that Dana could not see her daughter or be given any information about her. Dana was moved to another floor. Her desperate inquiries about her daughter were met with silence.

Over the next two weeks, Dana, distraught, in shock,

began to believe her family and the voices in her head that told her she could not raise this child alone, that it was best for both her and her daughter for the baby to be released to another family. Dana could hardly walk; she could not eat; she felt as though she had died. In her distress, she finally agreed.

Like Marianne, though, her story does not end here in loss. Dana's daughter was adopted by a family who surrounded her with love and attention. Mother and daughter were reunited twenty years later, a reunion that has planted each one irrevocably in the other's life.

These are some of the hardest stories I know. But even these stories of loss end in some kind of redemption. Perhaps the very hardest of all, where it is difficult to see any sign of grace or hope, happened recently in my own hometown and happens in hometowns everywhere. A sixteen-year-old girl, scared and shaking, told her parents she was pregnant. They coerced her into going to an abortion clinic. She did not want to end the baby's life, but she was given no choice. She lost her baby.

I want to say these stories of pain are rare, but that would not be the truth. The truth is that even within marriage, even within a relationship that feels solid, a pregnancy that suddenly appears in the midst of a normal life can sometimes lead to unexpected responses. Chris was happily married—until she became pregnant unexpectedly. Her husband did not support the pregnancy. When she refused to get an abortion, he became bitter toward her for carrying their child. She has no idea what the future holds for her and her marriage; she only knows that she loves this child.

Yet for every one of these women who told and then lost control over the life of her baby, there are far more experiences of women whose fears never became reality.

Rosa dreaded spilling the news that at age thirty-three she was pregnant, with no marriage or the father anywhere in sight. Her relationship with her own father, a doctor, was already troubled. His violent moods created a kick-me, beat-me, show-me-that-you-care kind of relationship between them. Rosa lived in fear of his rejection—he had already cut off all communication with one of her siblings. It was fear of his disapproval that had led her to abort her first pregnancy several years before. That abortion was the lowest point of her life. This time she would not abort.

She could not tell him to his face, though, so she wrote a letter. "I said, 'I know you're going to be real disappointed, but I don't care. I didn't plan this, but I always wanted a baby. It doesn't look like I'll ever get married. I'm going to have this baby anyway. I hope you can deal with it. I love you very much, but this is the way it is.'"

Her parents wrote back suggesting abortion, which cut Rosa deeply. Her father had always been adamantly against abortion. But he didn't reject her, as she feared. Neither did he reject the baby, as she had also feared. Grandson and grandfather came to love each other deeply.

Jill Rohrer also had plenty of reason to keep silent, plenty of reason to fear telling. Her father was a pastor. She had spent much of her life in church. That spring she had just graduated from a Christian college. She had been taught all her life that sleeping with a boyfriend was biblically wrong. And yet they had slept together on several occasions—Jill's attempt, she later realized, to hang on to him when he appeared to be losing interest in her. What would happen if she told her family? There would be such shame. Maybe her father would lose his church. Would her younger sisters, who had always looked up to her, even speak to her? And what about work? She had just landed a good teaching job in an elementary school—her first teaching position. What if the school administrators didn't approve of her unmarried and pregnant status? How could she look people in the eye, knowing she had violated so much of what she believed in?

Yet, of course, she knew she had to tell. At some point she recognized she didn't have much more to lose. Already she had distanced herself from her parents and her sisters, with whom she had always been close. She stopped going to church. At the last church service she had been to, Communion had been served. Jill, her face set, let the plate of bread and wine pass her by. At work she wore loose, flowing dresses, throwing up in the bathroom between classes. Finally the hiding—from her family, from her co-workers, from God—became too much. She chose a Friday night to drive home. Everyone would be there, she knew.

After dinner, as everyone got up to leave, Jill blurted out, "Uh, could you hold on for a second? I have something to tell all of you." One of her sisters got a big grin on her face and said, "Oh! You're going to get married!" Jill's face tensed and hardened. This was the very thing she desired most, but everything had gone awry. This man she had cared about was already backing out of any commitments to her and now to this baby. She knew he'd soon be gone entirely.

"Noooo," Jill drawled out, her head tilted. Then in a now-or-never rush, she blurted out, "I'm going to have a baby. I've been to the doctor, and I know for sure, and I'm really sorry." Then she just sat, waiting. Her father and mother sat frozen, her sisters sat unmoving—all with big eyes. Then in what seemed like a single move, both parents rushed to her side, offering comfort and support.

The people in her father's church were much the same. The next Sunday night as her father met with the deacons, gravely sharing the news, they responded with grace. "We want to support you completely. Don't leave the church over this, either you or Jill!" One man put it in perspective: "This is not a bad thing—this is a baby! There are a lot worse consequences to sexual activity than a baby."

For many, telling brings an end to the isolation and

loneliness of carrying the news alone. If circumstances make telling especially difficult, take a friend with you who can be calm and supportive. If you don't feel able to break the news in person, write a letter first, as Rosa did, or call. This is the part you are responsible for—letting the truth be known. The second part of telling—the response—is now their responsibility. If the response from your parents, your spouse, or your boyfriend is not supportive, there *are* others who will support you. There *are* others who care about this still-forming child, who may care about this new life even more than you do right now. Break your silence—let friends, siblings, relatives, or women at pregnancy centers help you and your baby. If you feel alone and don't know where to go for help, there are resources at the back of this book that can provide a starting point. And when you tell the people you trust, tell *all* the truth: "I am pregnant, and I didn't mean to be. This is very hard for me right now. I need your help." Even in a longtime marriage, I needed help. For those first weeks I felt lost, and no one knew it. Everyone assumed it was another pregnancy as normal until I dared to speak, to tell the whole truth, to cry on offered arms. Let others know you are lost, and they will begin to help you find the way.

Three

Heartbeat

You will be able to hear your baby's heartbeat

through a stethoscope this month.

Your baby has fingers, toes and soft nails.

By the end of this month of pregnancy,

he is four inches long

and weighs a little over an ounce.

—WWW.SUREBABY.COM

For you created my inmost being;

you knit me together in my mother's womb.

I praise you because I am fearfully

and wonderfully made.

—PSALM 139:13–14

I am in the doctor's office, a low gray building that overlooks an ocean inlet. I have been going to the same doctor for twenty-five years. The first time I met him he was wearing jeans and running shoes and introduced himself as Mark, and he has been Mark ever since. He delivered my first baby fourteen years ago. I am on the exam table, pulling the cloth they call a gown back over my knees and any other skin it will cover. I almost physically push away the feelings of invasion.

"Well, congratulations. You're definitely pregnant. You're eight to nine weeks right now, I'd say, at the beginning of your third month." Of course I knew this already, and so I say nothing. He is at the sink now, washing his hands, his back to me. He is maybe six or seven years older than I am, close enough that I think of him as a peer. He turns. "I thought you guys were done?" He looks at me quizzically, eyes crinkling into a smile. His son is in college, his daughter a senior in high school.

"We were. We are," I say without a hint of humor.

He looks at me carefully. Then, "Well, these things happen." He shrugs philosophically. "This is your—sixth?"

I nod.

He shakes his head knowingly, deciding how to react. "Wasn't your last one something of a surprise?"

"You could say that."

"How old is he now?"

"Abraham is fifteen months." And as I think of him, his joy and exuberance, how much light he has brought to our house, I smile for the first time since coming into the office.

"Oh, wow," he says, seeming slightly impressed. At what I'm not sure. Our stupidity? Our mistake? That we really goofed up here in producing another offspring? I am waiting to hear this in his voice, maybe in his words, and I'm ready to wince, but he is better than that.

"Well, you guys are busy," he says, nodding his head appreciatively. "Some people are just destined to pass their genes on." He lifts his eyebrows and smiles encouragingly as he says this. Okay, I decide. I'll take that. I organize a small smile in return.

"How old are you now?" He glances in the direction of my chart. "Are you forty-three?"

"Forty-four," I say flatly. "And I'll be forty-five when the baby is born." My voice is leaden. I know this is the outside edge of childbearing. And then the question I really came for: "Okay, so what's the miscarriage rate for my age?" I asked this when I first called, a week ago.

"Well, I wouldn't tell anyone about this pregnancy yet," he cautions. "The miscarriage rate at your age is 50 percent.

Wait until we hear the heartbeat before you tell anyone. Then the miscarriage rate drops to about 10 percent."

"Fifty percent?" I ask again. He nods. Did it have to be exactly 50 percent? What about 53 or 48 percent—something to tip the scales in one direction? What a tortuous number! Designed to rob the bearer of any certainty. Suddenly the other half of that number struck me; hope rose in my chest. Maybe this would all disappear in a few weeks! But I knew from my first miscarriage twenty years ago that it was hardly a happy event. What do I hope for—a new life or some kind of death?

Mark sees the confusion and worry on my face. "Come back in two to three weeks. The longer you wait, the surer we'll be to get a heartbeat. We'll have a good idea then of what's going to happen."

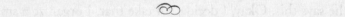

For many women this third month feels the longest. The shock has worn off. Now come the nausea, extreme fatigue, a sluggishness that won't sleep away. All signs of a new life coming, but it is still invisible. No maternity clothes yet, belly still pretty normal. But this month moves you toward something tangible. Soon, near the end of the month, you will go back to the doctor or midwife, and if the baby is there, you will hear the heartbeat.

It is a simple procedure to listen in on the uterus. A hand-held Doppler, that looks a little like a flashlight, is held against the abdomen, made slippery by a clear lubricant. The device is moved painlessly around the belly until the fetus is located by the heartbeat. The doctor or midwife visit is often brief and without incident, but the moment is powerful.

Theresa Peterson, unexpectedly pregnant at forty, lay on the couch in her living room with the midwife beside her. Her children were there, thirteen-year-old Charlie and eleven-year-old Meredith. Then there it was, a powerful little heartbeat filling the room. Charlie's and Meredith's eyes went wide, their eyebrows up, looking at one another, at their mother with amazement. They could not speak. Theresa drank in their wonder. It became real then: there was indeed a baby growing inside who would soon join their family.

But that three-month visit is not always without incident. Michele Gonzales found out she was pregnant in the basement bathroom of the state troopers building where her husband worked. They were going out to lunch together—a date! But the night before, Michele had complained again of exhaustion. She had plenty to make her tired—she had four children, she was nursing her youngest, who was nearly one, and she was homeschooling. For those reasons and more, they had decided four was all they could manage. They were taking measures to prevent another pregnancy, and permanent birth control was just around the corner. This winter they were all going on a family vacation to Hawaii, their first in five years. That night Lonnie remarked, offhand, "Gee, you're never this tired except when you're pregnant." Those words stabbed at Michele. The next day, the test. And the line. She stormed into her husband's office and threw the test on his desk, livid. He had no idea what this foreign object was and so began to examine it. Finally he looked up, realizing what it was. Michele started, "This is your fault! Why didn't you get the vasectomy! I even set up the appointment for you!" Mentally she raced through all it would mean: no more size-seven blue jeans; the Hawaii vacation—gone; now five children in an eleven-hundred-square-foot apartment; one more child to homeschool... Lonnie saw none of that, only that he would have another son or daughter.

The third month came—time for a routine checkup. Though her heart was not in any of this, Michele went dutifully. This time she would hear the heartbeat, the doctor told her. She lay on the table, her shirt up under her armpits, the Doppler on her already-expanding belly. Michele winced. She had worked hard to strengthen her abdominal muscles after her last pregnancy, and now—so soon gone again. As she waited for the familiar sound of static and the sure, steady beat of another heart, she thought of how many times she had done this before. But where was it—that familiar shump, shump? The doctor was still moving the Doppler around and would catch the slower beat of her heart, but nothing else. After several minutes he frowned ever so slightly, put the Doppler away, wiped the lubricant from Michele's belly, and calmly said it would be good to have an ultrasound.

Michele was not worried. She'd had several ultrasounds before, and all had confirmed her best hopes—normal, healthy babies, every one. But this time was different. Her husband was there, his first time ever to see one of his unborn children. The technician rolled the instrument around on her belly while Michele watched the screen. *There he is. Yes, it is a boy,* she noted. *Okay—two girls and three boys,* she silently recited without excitement. *But why is the technician so silent? Why doesn't he give me the usual travel monologue—"Here's the head. Here's the heart"?* She began to be alarmed. Something was wrong. And then she thought, *How could it be? I'm healthy. I take good care of my body. My children are all healthy.*

The technician called in the doctor, who came and finished the scan. Michele and Lonnie knew for certain something was wrong, though they could not tell it from the screen. Just as the doctor finished, he turned to them and told them that the baby was missing an umbilical artery. An older man with a curt manner, he laid out the worst-case scenario right then and there. "Without an adequate blood supply, the baby could have a cleft palate, a hair lip, urinary troubles, low birthweight…" He went on and on, listing every birth defect known, it seemed. Michele grabbed Lonnie's hand. She had seen this baby now; he was alive, but he could be suffering. Her heart almost hurt at this thought. What if he didn't survive? Would it be her fault for not wanting him? How would she live with that? *I have loved all my other babies. Surely I can love this one too,* she reasoned. *If he survives.* Her weight gain, their crowded house, the lost vacation—all that she dreaded began to diminish in importance.

The rest of the pregnancy Michele took special care to eat well and to get as much rest as she could. Because she lived in a remote area, every few weeks she flew four hours to the nearest neonatal hospital, where doctors carefully monitored the baby's progress. The shadow of anxiety never left, but she countered with prayer. She prayed for that baby more than she had prayed for anyone.

Levi was born three weeks early, small but healthy, without a single defect. He was not an easy baby, though. He did not sleep well, and he screamed with colic most of the evening hours. The nights walking him around the small room, her face dark with fatigue, Michele thought about the troubled pregnancy. *Why did all that happen?* She is certain that prayer made a difference in the outcome—maybe not just for Levi but for her as well. No, not a perfectly happy ending, as she paced the floor wearily in her larger-sized jeans, but it had turned out better than she had feared. *Maybe everything happened the way it did for my sake!* she thinks now. *I stopped thinking so much about myself and started thinking about him.*

For those who have had miscarriages before and those who are older, this is the month of breath holding. Ninety percent of all miscarriages occur during these weeks. For those struggling with infertility, for those desiring their first or another child, hope and prayer move in a single direction: *Please, Lord, oh please let this baby make it!* For the rest of us, it is much more complicated. What do you do during these weeks of waiting? How should you feel? What do you wish for, pray for? Should you emotionally invest in this child, make room in your life for someone who may yet lie in your arms? Or is this not a child at all, just a mass of cells that will glob into nothing and then leave in a bloody mess? And then, with every thought about the possibility of losing the baby, with every fleeting second of hope that the baby will not make it, there falls the immediate and heavier weight of guilt.

Unexpected pregnancy is like this—complicated, confusing. But moments of clarity come like handholds along the winding way.

Pam Tripp knows about all of this. Her story of unexpected pregnancy comes from the other end—from a ten-year struggle with secondary infertility. How strange that someone consumed for so long with desire for a child should struggle and nearly reject a surprise pregnancy. But Pam's story is echoed by others who have swung this wild pendulum. For her, too, the first moment of clarity centered around the heartbeat.

Pam and Chuck tried for years to have a baby. Finally, eleven years ago, Laura was born. Soon after, they began trying for another. They wanted Laura to have a sibling—a simple, ordinary desire. But it was not to be. They could conceive—the pregnancy tests read positive again and again—but each time, usually before the third month, a miscarriage. Two pregnancies brought Pam all the way through the third month to the exam table where the Doppler chugged with the engine of the heartbeat, but one week later or two, the baby was gone. Those two times it had been a boy. After seven years of this, Pam and Chuck made a decision: They could not bear these steep plunges from life to death; they would no longer try for another child. This decision brought an unexpected freedom to carry on with their lives.

Nearly three years later they took a ten-year-old foster son into their home. They grew to care deeply for him and began the adoption process, but it did not go through. Pam felt as if she'd had another miscarriage. How did she keep losing children?

Shortly after that loss they conceived again. Pam could

not believe it. She cried out to God, "Lord, what are you asking me to do? Do I have to go through the valley of the shadow of death—*again*?" She had no reason to hope; she already knew that God could let it happen over and over. Her life had gone on well since the earlier decision, taken on its own speed, picked up other ambitions and plans. She was going to return to school, take more classes in Web design and graphics, and open her own business. She would return to her other passion, quilting. She was done with babies and the confinement and isolation they brought. Her life was complete. Why was this happening now?

The weeks passed, bringing her to the doctor for the first fetal checkup. Because of her history, she was scheduled for an ultrasound instead of just the Doppler in the doctor's office. Pam felt numb. She did not want to go through this. Even if all was well at this point and the heartbeat was strong, she knew it didn't guarantee anything.

Laura was with them, although Pam had mixed feelings about pulling her daughter into a story with a tragic ending. She reasoned that if the baby didn't live, Laura would at least see her brother or sister and know he or she had been real.

The ultrasound could not have been more exciting. They saw the fetus—a girl—spinning, bouncing, jumping around like a hyperactive astronaut. Pam and Chuck and Laura smiled and laughed, and for the first time, Pam felt a spark of hope. She was able to release the moment and think, *Even if we don't get to have this child, we have seen her alive and well.*

This story did not have a tragic ending. Pam never trusted the pregnancy or her body. She did not buy a stitch of clothing or any other baby item until Sarah was born. But the pregnancy she did not expect or want became a welcomed daughter. The first moment of that becoming was there in the radiology room.

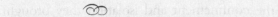

What will you feel when you hear the heartbeat for the first time? My own three weeks between clinic visits passed in slow motion when I was pregnant with Micah. And then the day—May 18, a Tuesday. I knew what this visit was all about. It was about finding out whether I got my life back, restored to me as it was, or whether I would be home again, my life utterly changed. Either way, it meant freedom from the 50 percent statistic that held me, tyrannically, in suspension. I had reasoned all this out long before the short trip to the clinic.

I entered the exam room; Duncan was with me. The pull of clean paper over the exam table, the squirt of cold lubricant on my belly, the flinch, the wait as the instrument rounded my abdomen, the sound of static, then the beat of my own heart—a slow, low pulsing—and then there, in the lower left, a sudden shug, shug erupted from the Doppler. There it was—a life! My eyes widened in shock as if I had never heard another's heartbeat inside my own body. I looked at Duncan, my face asking, *Do you hear it?* For the first time since the test, I felt a surge of emotions. *Listen to it! So strong, so fast, so purposeful. How has something so perfectly made, so full of purpose, so full of life—how has this been made without our permission, without our intent?* And yet it has.

Pam, Michele, Theresa, I, and so many others still remember that moment: a tiny creature deep within us, just two inches long, has a heartbeat that fills the room. And suddenly this unintended pregnancy, this complication, this interruption becomes—a life.

The Second Trimester

Four

Showing

In this month the back straightens, hands and feet
are well-formed...finger closure is possible.
Reflexes become more active as muscle maturation continues.
The fetus begins to stir and so thrust out arms and legs
in movements readily perceived by the mother.
—WWW.CHILDDEVELOPMENTINFO.COM

Before I was born the LORD called me;
from my birth he has made mention of my name....
He said to me, "You are my servant...
in whom I will display my splendor."
—ISAIAH 49:1, 3

I am going to a reception tonight. What will I wear? I am not ready to announce my pregnancy, so maternity clothes are out, camouflage is in. I want to delay the inevitable, the callousness and sometimes cruelty of acquaintances. Even good friends and colleagues can say the stupidest things to a pregnant woman. After I revealed my last pregnancy to an administrator at the university—speaking quietly with humility and embarrassment—he looked at me open-mouthed, then replied, "This is your, what—ninth or tenth?" After that same pregnancy, one woman, an attorney I barely knew who had one child, came up to me on a street corner and patted my abdomen (which was considerably flatter than hers), saying, "What? Aren't you pregnant? Every time I see you you're pregnant!" She then draped her arm around my shoulders in a familiar and conspiratorial manner, offering in a stage whisper to enlighten me on the cause of such events. Her actions and words have been repeated by countless others, all of whom surely—I am choosing to believe—do not intend to be foolish and hurtful. But I am not ready to face all of this yet. I need to do what Michael Schwarz did the day she learned of her pregnancy: she began to formulate answers to the questions and comments she knew were coming. "I know Sarah's going to say to me after church, 'Don't you know how that happens?' I'm going to say back, 'No, Sarah, maybe you can explain to me how sperm gets by a condom.'"

I will work on preparing some answers later. For now, I continue the search, pulling through the dresses and skirts in my closet, trying on the burgundy floral skirt with the elastic waist—no, too tight. What about the olive green slacks with the stretchy waist? I pull them on, standing in front of the mirror as they lift up and over and—the two sides of the zipper are inches apart. I sigh, turn, and look at my profile: only four months along, and a definite pooch, bigger than previous pregnancies. This is hardly a surprise; I know it works like this. Muscles lose their tone, their stretch and flexibility, but even so, I am mad at myself: I have gained too much weight already. I know in one part of my brain that this extra is completely justified, that this bulge in my abdomen is a human being, but I am not ready to surrender my body to another.

After Abraham was born, it took a full year to squeeze back into my jeans. A year of breast-feeding, exercising, being careful about what I ate. A year of hard work to regain enough of a waist to snap those buttons closed. I could hardly breathe or move, but little matter—they were on! I stood in front of the mirror feeling absurdly grateful, as if a gift had been given to me: I had not completely lost my body after all.

Every pregnancy felt perilous, as though stepping off a cliff. Where would I land? Would I recognize myself after the fall? Or would I just collect the pieces of my flesh, slap them back together as best I could, and chalk it up to the cost of another baby? When I stood in those ridiculously tight jeans, I was certain I had made it. We would have no more children, which meant I had survived my five pregnancies, and my recognizable body was back—the prodigal returns!

It was only four weeks after that celebratory moment that the news of another pregnancy broke. I wrote this in my journal:

I am going to burn my closet, all those clothes I JUST got back into after the last pregnancy. Leggings again, stretch pants, accordion-pleated tops, billowing sails.... I will strangle myself with anything containing spandex, clothes that affix no boundary upon my body. Will I survive it all again or just inflate like a dirigible, never to find my bones again, never to walk light and small upon this earth?? No, I won't gain weight this time. Not a pound. I'll stop eating. I'll starve myself. I can't do it again!

I am not proud of any of this. I am not proud of this obsession with body, with the number on the label of every piece of clothing that tells whether you pass the test or not, as though these numbers define you, explain you. *Am I really this superficial?* I wonder. *Where is my faith? Where are intellect and reason and all I know to be true about mind and body and spirit? That authentic beauty is internal. That the body is temporary and untrustworthy. That this weight gain and reshaping of the body are a small cost for giving life to another...* Yet I know I am not alone. In my interviews I heard the same things:

> "I was a size six until the pregnancy. I wondered if I would ever be that size again."

> "I had just lost twenty pounds—and I knew all that was gone. I was going to have to work off those twenty pounds again."

> "I had lost all my weight from my last pregnancy and was down to a size seven again. I had worked so hard, going to a weightroom, working on my muscles...and now I'm pregnant again?"

Pregnancy chat rooms are full of these anxieties, of women in the middle of their pregnancies comparing their weight:

"I'm at fifteen weeks and have gained twelve pounds already. Is this too much?"

"I'm thirteen weeks pregnant and am hungry all the time. I've already gained eight pounds, which is more than my doctor says I need. I'm feeling fat already. Should I cut back?"

"I'm at twenty-five weeks, and I've gained twenty-two pounds. I feel enormous! Is there anyone out there who has gained as much as me?"

Every woman facing pregnancy deals with this, but for those who come to pregnancy unprepared and unwilling, it can be even harder to submit to these changes in our bodies that may feel like changes to the very core of our selves. I cannot explain it completely, why the size we wear matters so much to who we feel ourselves to be. And since Hollywood recently discovered pregnancy, the standard has risen. Madonna, Gwyneth Paltrow, Julia Roberts, and others parade their perfect, pregnant bodies on magazine covers, late-night television, not an extra pound gained. Soon after the baby is born, they are back in belly shirts, abdomens flat, sexy, and unchanged. Who can compete? Even though we know their breezy after-pregnancy shape is the result of their own obsession with their looks and grueling daily workouts with personal trainers and in-home professional chefs, we still feel the pressure.

These fears about our bodies are not just harmless anxieties. When a pregnancy is unintended, women and the babies they carry are at higher risk. The mother is less likely to seek thorough prenatal care; she is more likely to continue drinking alcohol and smoking; a higher percentage of babies are born at a lower birth weight.[5] Jana expressed some of the feelings behind these risks: "I did go to the doctor, but I didn't really care what I ate. I ate whatever I wanted—junk food, cookies, whatever I felt like. I didn't take my vitamins—I didn't care. I was angry at God."

As I looked at the statistics and heard these words from Jana and others, I knew that harm to the baby would be the worst of everything. Though it feels as if the pregnancy will last forever, you know it will not. But if care is not taken during the pregnancy, the birth may be harder, and there is a higher chance that the child who comes may require more care than usual, possibly even for a lifetime. Who could live with this? Especially if it were preventable.

Shortly into my pregnancy with Micah, I gave up on my hysterical vow not to gain weight. Soon thereafter I gave up on the whole pregnancy-by-numbers game. I stopped weighing myself. Even at the doctor's, I wouldn't let them tell me my weight. No more numbers that were like scores to tell me if I was winning or losing. I ate healthy food—along with a hot fudge sundae a few times a week—exercised as much as I could, and let that be enough.

Others have come to the same conclusion. Lisa, pregnant now for the seventh time, knows that the hardest time for her is around the fourth month. "That's when I feel the most self-conscious. In my first two pregnancies, I would just feel like I was getting fat. My clothes didn't fit anymore, but maternity clothes were too big. That awkward stage. But later, when I really look pregnant, I don't care as much. I'm not going to eat extravagantly, you know, McDonald's every day, but I'm not going to diet. I just try to eat good food, make sure the baby's growing and is healthy, and worry about the weight later. I look at other women who are pregnant, and I don't think they look fat! They're just pregnant!"

In fact, pregnant women often have higher body-image satisfaction than nonpregnant women. Angela, pregnant at sixteen, felt this way.

> When [I] started to show, and the first time I felt it
> kick, I thought, "Wow!" It was amazing to feel some-
> thing moving inside of me and know that I made
> that. I loved the feeling when the baby kicked. I liked
> being pregnant. My hair was a lot healthier, and my
> skin was really good. I liked my stomach, how it felt,
> how it looked in clothes. It's so comfortable when
> you're sleeping, you can rest your arm on your big

stomach. The baby was huge, my stomach was really big. Everybody pays attention to you and wants to touch your stomach. It was a nice feeling.[6]

There *are* good things in this, we tell ourselves, and we know it is true. We can eat food without counting every calorie. We can dress comfortably, freed from the cultural demand that we look like *Vogue* models. Michael went out and "spent a fortune," she told me, on new maternity clothes, which helped her feel better about how she looked. We can exercise, which raises the "feel good" endorphins in the brain and keeps muscles fit and toned for labor and afterward.

In fact, studies show that women who exercise report a greater sense of satisfaction with their bodies and their pregnancies. Katrina Neff is a good example of this. In her first pregnancy, she gained a lot of weight and started to get edema, swelling in her legs. With a family history of circulatory problems, Katrina was scared and started walking. She walked a half hour a day at first, then an hour, even longer on some days, until she was hiking up long hills easily. Her weight stabilized, her energy increased, and her sleep was longer and deeper. She was hooked. In succeeding pregnancies, Katrina made sure, no matter how busy she was, to make time for walking. After six children, Katrina today weighs the same as when she was first married.

What about after the pregnancy? The other half of the fear is wondering, if we make it through a healthy pregnancy, will we be able to take off the weight after the baby is born? Is there Life After Birth? The news from that shore is the same as from every shore, it seems: individual to every woman. Some women, like Katrina and Lisa, have stories of quick weight loss with little change to their bodies. Others have stories of weight that finally budged after a year, maybe two or even three, but it happened. For others, the changes from pregnancy last longer.

Carol Nelson was thirty-nine when her last child, Annie, was born. Annie was her sixth. Carol had done well with her other kids—losing all her pregnancy weight within four or five months. She was so happy, so thankful to get her body back each time. Then this surprise pregnancy. Carol gained only twenty-six pounds during the pregnancy, but after the birth—a planned C-section—the weight just wouldn't move.

> After I had her, I waited and waited for the weight to start coming off, but it wouldn't. I would exercise, diet—nothing worked. I was so aware of my body, thinking that I would never be able to wear a bathing suit again. Not that anyone would look anyway. But I just don't want to stand in front of the mirror and think, *That's gross!* It's been seven years since she was

born. I'm still living with being thirty pounds over-weight.

Even so, I realize that losing weight is not the most important thing in my life. It's not going to make me a better person; it's not going to affect the way I react or love or correct my children, or the way that I live my life for the Lord. In the last couple of years I realized my relationship with the Lord is the most important thing. And as I focus on that, he'll help me with the self-discipline to not let myself go. My physical appearance is not the most important thing. It's not all about me!

I, too, discovered something about this. Three months after Micah's arrival I sat on a warm tropical beach swarming with spring breakers. So many bodies on display: buttocks, breasts, tightly ripped abs, whittled waists, creamy brown skin... I began to envy all these body parts so other than my own. I still carried fifteen extra pounds from the pregnancy, and I knew I wouldn't lose them all until I stopped nursing, eight months away. Even then, maybe I still wouldn't. I was ready for a furious envy session when Micah started fussing. Without a thought, I pulled him to me, lifted my shirt, and began to feed him, settling into the hot sand with the languor of nursing. Now, from this perspective, baby at my breast, legs tented, I looked again at all those parading young women. I felt stronger than them, wiser, more capable. Yes, they had flat bellies and firm, jiggling breasts, but I could do better. My belly had created *children*! My breasts not only looked good, but they actually *worked.* They *fed* people!

On the other side now of my final pregnancy, I can report that I did, finally, get back into the jeans I thought I would burn in memoriam for my lost body. It *is* possible—remember this. But who can promise that for someone else? If it does not happen, there are adjustments to make. There are compensations. Some so great they can hardly be measured or even described. One night near Christmas we went to visit my parents-in-law. Abraham, eighteen months old, took his usual spot on Grandpa's lap, but as the evening progressed, Abraham climbed up higher and fell asleep on his chest. DeWitt, at eighty-six, had weathered strokes, a heart attack, and cancer. His doctor had advised on more than one occasion to let nature take its course, but DeWitt rallied and surprised us all by recovering each time. Through all the hospital visits, it was Abraham's baby face that lit DeWitt's eyes the brightest. That night Abraham's softness pooled on DeWitt's chest and belly, his mouth open against his grandfather's neck, breathing lightly. DeWitt was almost sleeping now too, his stiff right hand supporting Abraham's bottom, his own lips puffing out with each breath. I looked at these two resting together, one who should have died several times over and the other who, by human intent, would not be living at all. Who are we to decide who lives and dies? And the number on the tag inside my jeans—yes, it was a higher number because of this sleeping baby, but what did that have to do with anything that mattered? It is part of the cost of life, the stretching of our bodies and lives to nourish another. Years ago it was me inside, stretching my mother's body. All our mothers made room for us. We will do the same.

Five

Finding Out

By the end of the fifth month, the activity of this
8- to 10-inch fetus is strong enough to be felt
by its mother. Soft downy lanugo covers its body;
hair begins to grow on its head; brows and white eyelashes
appear. A protective vernix coating covers the fetus.
—*WHAT TO EXPECT WHEN YOU'RE EXPECTING*

My frame was not hidden from you
when I was made in the secret place.
When I was woven together in the depths of the earth,
your eyes saw my unformed body. All the days
ordained for me were written in your book
before one of them came to be.
—PSALM 139:15–16

The fifth month. My wardrobe is all stretch and pleats now. I've given up any pretense of concealing my figure. Anyone who looks knows. But just as this pregnancy becomes more public, I have the chance to look inside, to peer into the dark of my womb and learn something of the secret growing there. Most doctors recommend an amniocentesis for all of us over thirty-five, because the statistics for fetal abnormalities begin to increase with our age. This is the month the test is usually done. It's not a complicated procedure, but it requires delicacy. With an ultrasound providing the visual window, the doctor slowly inserts a needle into the belly, staying clear of the baby, and draws fluid out, usually painlessly. The fluid contains minute particles of the fetus's DNA, enough to detect gender and certain conditions: Down syndrome, cystic fibrosis, and others.

When pregnant with my fourth child at age thirty-seven, I was offered this test and others, but I refused them. I was healthy, fit, ate the right foods, and had few risk factors. I was not worried about either defects or gender then and decided simply to trust that the pregnancy would unfold as it should. For the last two pregnancies I chose the amniocentesis. The numbers were not good for me; the chances for abnormalities given my "advanced maternal age" were far too close for comfort. In fact, the chart listing these numbers ended with my age—forty-five. There I was, at the bottom of the chart, on the far edge of childbearing. I felt a great urgency to know anything I could—health, size, number of toes, full beating heart, nail-biter or thumb-sucker, girl or boy... Whatever the answer, whatever was found, I would at least know and have time to prepare. I had had enough surprises.

All of us in these pages who had an ultrasound or amnio came away from that doctor's visit changed—from knowing nothing about the child within us to knowing something. Sometimes that knowledge lightened the load; sometimes it did not. Shoshana experienced both. Her first ultrasound in her first pregnancy revealed a baby girl with a thickened neck fold, a possible sign of Down syndrome. If that wasn't enough, a later ultrasound confirmed what they feared, that 50 percent of her placenta had separated from the wall of her uterus. The doctors urged her to abort, telling her with certainty in their voices that this baby girl would have special needs all her life. Shoshana would not consider it. She would not even have an amniocentesis. "I told them I just had to have faith that things would turn out okay." Amazingly, her daughter was born healthy and normal. But her story continues.

With three girls now—their baby and Jon's two daughters from a previous marriage, the eldest with cerebral palsy—Shoshana and Jon decided that their cups were overflowing. Jon had always wanted a son, but after the last high-risk pregnancy and with the stress and frequent medical emergencies with their oldest, they agreed they didn't have the resources; it wouldn't be fair to their family to add another child. As the youngest turned three, plans were made for a vasectomy to be done as soon as Jon came back from his National Guard Reserve training. While he was away, Shoshana discovered she was pregnant.

"When I saw the test was positive, I thought, *What is this?* It was a week before my husband was to get home. A week to get more angry at him that he hadn't gone in [for the vasectomy] yet! This can't be happening! When you make the decision to be done—and for good reasons—and then have that decision changed on you, you're upset, angry. *God, you're making me go back on that decision!*"

Shoshana had reasons to be upset. Her youngest had learned to walk in hospital corridors during long stays with Shoshana's oldest daughter. She didn't want to do that again, to raise another baby while dashing in and out of hospitals. And she was sure it was going to be another girl, "another shot of hormones." Jon was certain too. They found it difficult to summon up excitement about adding another female to their household.

By the fifth month another ultrasound was scheduled because of Shoshana's last high-risk pregnancy. She agreed to it, but nothing more—no amniocentesis, no multiple-marker screening test, no alpha-fetoprotein test. She did not want to lurch from test to test as she had done before, everything cast in a pall of worry. As Shoshana lay on the table, all three of her girls around her, the technician spotted the telltale body part. Not a neck fold, but a penis. "It's a boy!" he announced, watching the screen. The girls laughed with excitement. Shoshana felt a sudden and unexpected release—a boy! Now that was something new! In a surge of exhilaration she reached up and high-fived the technician, who was grinning at their delight. She couldn't wait to tell Jon. It made a difference for both of them. The pregnancy went by faster; Shoshana and Jon now felt anticipation for the new child.

Trisha Pruitt lived in a household of boys: she had four, the eldest just graduating from high school, the youngest about to enter first grade. Their home was a refuge not only for her boys but for their friends as well. Trisha also ran a day care during working hours to help support the family. There was not a moment of the day when the house was not full of children—mostly boys—shouting, racing down the halls, shaking the floors with trampoline jumps on the beds.

Trisha knew the importance of letting her boys release their physical energy, but it was exhausting, the sheer testosterone of it all.

Other factors complicated her days. Chris, her second son, had developed a heart condition and was home often, resting, unable to go to school. The youngest, Joey, age six, who had been born prematurely, had taken Trisha and Steve through a number of health issues.

They had both always wanted a girl, but the thought of another baby and the potential for health problems petrified them. Their dinner table was more than full; their family was complete. Everyone was moving forward. They had dispensed with the thought of another baby years ago. Besides, Trisha reasoned, she knew that if she had another, it would be a boy. Five boys! Just the thought of it was overwhelming.

When the pregnancy test read positive, Trisha was in denial for days, even weeks. Like so many of us, she was angry, grief stricken, anxious. She loved her boys fiercely, but the thought of another boy to add to her daily pandemonium was too much. Steve, with father's intuition, was sure it was a girl. Trisha almost did not dare to hope, but her hopes were confirmed with an ultrasound and amniocentesis.

"When they told me it was a girl, I started crying. I cried and cried. I had held off buying anything for the baby until I knew, but then I went and started shopping right away for girl stuff. It was like a dream. It just instantly made the rest of the pregnancy easier."

∽

Finding out the sex of this new child can change everything.

My first amnio and ultrasound, in the first unplanned pregnancy, confirmed what I had already told myself—yes, it was another boy. I nodded slowly when the technician gave the news. I was relieved to know now. I did not want to feed hopes for a girl for nine months, creating a plump little butterball of a dream daughter only to greet an entirely other person on the delivery table.

That known, what about the rest, what about the more significant news: Is he healthy? Are the measurements right? What's been going on in there these last five months while I've been busy out here on the other side of my skin? I watched intently as the wand circled my belly. There he was. I watched this minute person as he somersaulted, treaded water, mooned us with his tiny bottom, then scooted out of the way of the invading needle. I was as amazed as in my first pregnancy. Already so alive. *Already so much has developed without me,* I thought guiltily.

In other pregnancies it had been different. I had followed the pregnancy books' week-to-week diary of development as if the fetus's life depended upon it. *This week the fingernails form, the eyelids grow. This week some babies begin to suck their thumbs; lanugo, tiny hairs all over the body, begins to form this week...* I had traced the cell-on-cell creation of each child, thinking that to know was somehow to participate in, to agree with, to contribute to the making of this person. But I hadn't done that this time. And there he was, just as alive and perfect as any baby could be. I could fight it, or I could recognize how much bigger than me all this was.

∞

The second time I had an amnio and ultrasound, in the second unexpected pregnancy, it was harder. The world shifted and moved back again. It was July. All the way to the clinic from my small island, throughout two flights, I was quiet, knowing this last piece of the puzzle would be found. After birthing four boys in a row, I had a secret gnawing excitement that perhaps *this* last time it would be a girl, that perhaps this surprise was a gift of another kind. I knew all about boys. Like Trisha, my house and my life marinated in all stages of boyness. Maybe, as with Trisha and Shoshana, this was something different. And wouldn't that be so sweet of God to complete our family this way? Though it had hardly been my choice, this would be such quick redemption for this late-in-life pregnancy. Duncan felt the same. He loved his one daughter so much that he had joked and sparred with me for years after our first four were born and our family was complete. "If you knew that the next one would be a girl, wouldn't you have one more?" I could almost say yes to that, could almost feel myself yielding, but I answered the same every time: "If we had another one, I promise you, it would be a boy."

I thought of all this as I lay flat on the exam table, the white paper beneath me bunching and crumpling as I wiggled to get comfortable. I hoped to be proven a false prophet, to be wrong about my own ringing pronouncement. I would soon know. I looked up at the screen positioned overhead, like a television in hospital rooms. The technician squeezed the cold lubricant onto my belly, the wand made contact, and the screen overhead came alive. I was eyes only, looking to see who had entered my world with such determination. The head, yes, the arms, those feet, treading water so expertly, and then… "Oh, I see a little pee-pee," she said, in a happy, condescending voice. I looked intently, following her eyes. Yes, there it was. The session went on and on, with her cheerful narration of every body part and movement, but I was no longer watching. I wanted to leave; I wanted to find a quiet place to let this last desire go, my idea of who this was supposed to be. There was so much letting go these days. *What would be left of my life?* I wondered, deep in pity.

It did not feel like self-pity, though, until several days later when I learned that the very day I saw and mourned the coming of another son, my good friends Craig and Lisa lost their infant son, Peter, to SIDS. Just six months old, nearly the same number of weeks as my baby within my womb.

At the funeral, the pews of the church full, I sat cradling

my hands over my belly, the son I still carried, while sobbing for the son they had lost. In the face of this death, I knew at the deepest level possible that birth and the coming of any new life was *not* death. It felt like it at times, all the giving up of self, the loss of dreams and plans, the erosion of the most basic human needs—sleep, food, rest—but it was *not* dying. Even the surprise children who arrive with special needs. I realized I was one of the lucky ones. There's a cradle in the nursery instead of a casket at the front of the church. Each one of us in this book has been asked to bring forth and love and raise another life. Boy or girl, healthy or needy, how much does this matter? This is not death.

    Please, let me remember this.

Six

Starting Over

The fetus weighs about 3 pounds now and is approximately
16 inches long. The skin is red and wrinkled.... The baby
has virtually filled all the available space in the uterus....
Your baby's heartbeat speeds up when you speak
and he or she can recognize your voice after birth.

—*THE COMPLETE BOOK OF PREGNANCY*
AND CHILDBIRTH

At that time the disciples came to Jesus and asked,
"Who is the greatest in the kingdom of heaven?"
He called a little child and had him stand among them.
And he said: "I tell you the truth, unless you change and
become like little children, you will never enter the kingdom
of heaven. Therefore, whoever humbles himself
like this child is the greatest in the kingdom of heaven."

—MATTHEW 18:1–4

T he last month of the second trimester. The pregnancy is more than halfway over.

After my fourth child was born, I felt a sense of completion. I also felt besieged with four children under the age of seven. But our house was full; our family was done. Elisha was the beautiful bow atop our family package. When he turned two and graduated from the church nursery to a real classroom—to the twos and threes down the hall—I felt a quiet thrill. No more babies, no more nursery, no more nursery duty for me. I felt as though I, too, had been promoted. Though our home life was boisterous and chaotic, I knew we were moving forward. Just six more months of diapers, then preschool, then kindergarten... I could cheerfully tick off the sequence and advancement on my fingers. Nearly every Sunday as I walked past the church nursery door, I felt it again—a sense of relief, the joy of graduating beyond the inarticulate and incessant needs of infants. Now I could grow up too, follow my children along as they climbed through each grade, ever upward!

Three years later. My eldest was twelve, finishing her

seventh-grade year; Elisha was five, just finishing kindergarten. We were a few months away from all four children
attending school together, a few months away from our release from twelve years of managing, arranging, and maneu-
vering within the complex world of part-time childcare. I
was elated. And it wasn't any too soon. I was forty-two, a
thoroughly middle-aged age, one that I felt deserved this
upward mobility. I envisioned my husband and myself as
mountain climbers—we had scaled the rockiest part of the
trail and were now moving toward smoother, higher terrain.

And then. All movement stopped. I was arrested mid-
climb and returned to an all-too-familiar place, a place completely physical. I was back to tending a body with nausea,
back to fighting its demands for sleep, back to nights without any sleep. I would soon be returned to feedings on
demand—my body once more a milk machine—to diapers,
to the upending of every trash can and sugar canister, to oat-
meal on the floor and patches of spit-up on my shoulder for
two more years. Back to the start of the trail, the bottom of
the mountain, square one. Starting over.

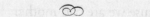

Most of us in this book cried when we discovered ourselves
pregnant. Many of us cried for this reason: we had been
there already. We counted ourselves survivors of it all—the

joy, the intensity, the loss of private space, the density of squirming little bodies all over ours, VeggieTales cakes, Thomas the Tank Engine birthday parties, the nursery rhymes sung while changing diapers, "Eensy-weensy Spider" in the car, seizing every moment to fill with language, learning, song. And from years of all this, emerge these children—whole, full, loud, bouncy, good kids. We stand back and wipe the sweat from our brows, amazed at who our children are becoming, wondrous at their strength given the fragility of our mothering. We are glad we did it all and wonder how we did it all. Where did the energy come from? We look at young mothers with their babies and toddlers in the grocery store, feeling empathy when the baby screams, when the brothers fight in the cart. And we smile with relief—Yup. Been there. Poor woman. I'm so glad it's not me anymore. If we are honest at all, there is also a certain smugness—we're a little more adult than she is, now that we don't have to bend so far to the ground. We walk upright most of the time.

Then, from that high plane, we are seized, arrested, and returned to it all. We cried—some for days, some for weeks—not because we are bad mothers but because we are good mothers, and we knew all it would take to be good mothers again.

Anna was forty-three, her husband fifty-two, when she found herself pregnant. Her daughter, who had been homeschooled most of her life, was graduating from high school; her son was eleven. Like the others, Anna felt anxious about beginning motherhood again, about all she would lose and give up and all she would have to do once more. The pregnancy alone was a huge hurdle. She had been sick, nearly bedridden, for each of her two previous pregnancies. Now this one. Yes, like the others it kept her in a constant state of nausea. Anna had to force herself to eat and had to stay close to the bathroom at all hours. She could no longer cook. Even caring for her family was a struggle.

Teresa Carlson raised her two girls in the middle of New York City, mostly as a single parent. She carried her daughters down the crowded city sidewalks, maneuvered through the difficulties of living in the city with two small children with little help. It was hard, but she was young, in her twenties, and she knew this part of her life would be done by the time she was forty. But no. Fifteen years later she was newly married—and pregnant. Her plans for retirement with her new husband and their move to a warmer climate for his arthritis were gone. Another child to raise instead. Teresa was back to a state of dependency she did not want.

Crystal Thomas did not want to start over, even though her other two children were still young; her elder daughter was nine, the younger, five. "I was scared," she admitted. "The two girls were such close friends. How would another baby affect them? We felt so complete as a family." So complete, in fact, that her husband had a vasectomy. That was in March. In April, Crystal was pregnant. "I felt really guilty that I wasn't joyful about another child. Here I was established with a house, a teaching job, a family, and I wasn't excited about gaining weight, about going through diapers again. When Sadie was potty training, I was celebrating—Yea! No more diapers! The whole time I was pregnant I only thought of the sleepless nights that were coming, the difficulties of nursing. I didn't embrace nursing; it was always so hard on me. It all felt like giant steps backward."

This is where most of us started and even stayed throughout the pregnancy. But I am here to say that the reports from the other side about Starting Over are hopeful and good. Like the other women here, I discovered I was wrong about some of my fears. Returning to pregnancy and infancy after a long absence, or even a short one, is often not the same experience. You may not be returning to what you think you already know. There are differences and changes coming that you cannot imagine now.

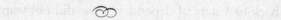

The stories these women tell after the arrival of their babies may read like a fairy tale or wishful thinking. I know you are not there now. But listen and believe that these words are true for these women—and allow the possibility that someday you may be able to speak the same.

For Anna, the birth of her daughter freed her from the nausea that virtually immobilized her throughout the pregnancy. She felt an immense freedom and renewed strength to move around, to enjoy food again, and to care for her new daughter. Even over the phone, I hear the calm in her voice. "I'm a better mother this time around. I know what's important. I'm not jumping up every minute to clean the house or work on my music, like I did with my other two. This is my last baby—ever. I'm just enjoying her, knowing this is the most important thing I can do."

Crystal, telling me about Gracie, now seventeen months old, doesn't talk about the messes Gracie makes in the cupboards, the sleep Crystal loses at night tending her, the work of juggling another child with a full-time job. This is not part of the report. She tells me instead about how she has changed and what Gracie has returned to her family's life. "I haven't worried about Gracie like I did with the others. I don't run to wash off the pacifier if it falls on the floor. She is a very important part of our family, she is such a joy, but the whole world doesn't revolve around her. I have a whole different perspective this time around. I had forgotten how fun it is when they discover the world. When I was pregnant, I didn't remember those things. I let my fears rob me of the joy I should have felt. I thought of all the hard things instead of all the good things—how fun it is to watch her play, to see her take her first steps, to run around the house with the older girls."

Ten months after Christian was born, Teresa found the reality of raising one more child much different than she expected. "I'm doing things completely differently than I did before. We moved to a rural community, where I have lots of support. I'm older and I have more patience. We know what we want and don't want for our son. I'm seeing the importance of having a complete family unit—of Christian having a dad. We have him sleep with us, and when he's done nursing, he'll just turn around and throw himself on his dad and hold his dad. I'm seeing the truth of the scripture that children are our heritage and our blessing from the Lord. I didn't think about those things when I was young. It's like we have another chance!"

Yes, you are starting over, but much has changed. *You* have changed, learned, and grown, even since the beginning of this pregnancy. You are wiser, smarter, more efficient than when you birthed your other children. Your other children are older. And most of all, a new person is coming whom you have never met. This is someone you have never held, never sung to, never nursed, never swaddled in fleece blankets, never taught to hold a spoon, never tucked in at night. No matter how many times you have done it before, you have never done it with this child. You are Starting Over— for the first time.

∞

Soon after Abraham was born, I was back in the church nursery, in the rocking chair with someone else's infant on my shoulder, Abraham sleeping contentedly in his carrier at my feet. I was fatigued from the two feedings in the night, and I was missing the church service, which I desperately needed, but I had signed up to serve in the nursery the month of February. During that month I thought back to the pregnancy, how I was doing now the very thing I feared and resented. No more waltzing past the gated nursery door. I was back within its confines, not only caring for my baby, but wiping other babies' spittle off my shoulder, rocking the fussy ones in the rocking chair, patting bottoms, changing other babies' messy diapers. But I did not feel defeated, nor did I feel resigned or resentful.

During that time in the nursery, I began to examine myself, to challenge my ideas of progress and success. I had always envisioned life as a graph, with a clear line that marched steadily through time, angling neatly upward toward the other side of the paper. This is how our lives are to look and feel: continual upward or forward movement as we strive toward growth, learning, advancement. It's a one-way path; a staircase to heaven; the corporate, professional, and social ladder angling to the roof. Promotion, maturity, knowledge, achievement. Child rearing graphed the same, I was sure. The whole process, from conception to adulthood, is marked by distinct, measurable stages, from the newborn who must be fed three times a night soon progressing to one feeding a night, then to none. Then the move from diapers to underwear, to the toddler dressing himself, on to the first day of school. The stages carry us along like the measured steps of a staircase toward graduation, the final launch to independence.

One of the first things I thought of when I discovered I was pregnant was how old I would be when that baby graduated from high school. I mentioned this to several friends in the same breath as announcing my pregnancy. "Would you believe I'm pregnant? And I'll be sixty-one when this baby graduates." And then two years later, when pregnant again, the updated version was, "And I'll be sixty-three when this baby graduates." I made this announcement looking for sympathy, knowing how many others chart their life course with a graph similar to mine. They would understand—and they did. They shook their heads in condolence, which confirmed what I already knew: my husband and I had ruined our life graph. Right in the middle the line now plunged, nearly touching the base of the chart. This meant failure, of course.

I suspected, though, instinctively and theologically, that something was wrong with this idea. I came to realize how thoroughly and how unconsciously I had absorbed the notion that there was an expiration date to parenting, that somehow at the end and top of the graphed line we could graduate to complete freedom, to release from all responsibility. Raise your children, sacrifice, devote yourselves to their well-being while they're under your roof, and when they're gone, you're done! Buy the Harley, go to Europe, collect shells on the beach, tour in the Winnebago. You've put in your time—this is *your* time. Do as you please.

Not everyone lives this way. I thought of women like Crystal and Rene, both mothers of surprise children who started over with all the attendant fears, all the wondering about whether they could return to caring for an infant again. They had both served as foster parents to dozens of children before their last baby was born. And even while their surprise child crawls at their feet, each told me of her plans to finish off the upstairs, to move to a larger house so she can have foster children again. To care for more children in need.

In that rocking chair, surrounded by babies—one screaming, two tussling, a few sleeping, two chasing a ball—I remembered a scene from the New Testament. The disciples are gathered around Jesus, and they have an important question. They all want to know: "Who is the greatest in the kingdom of heaven?" They ask not altogether innocently. They know the answer. They are, of course. Hadn't Jesus handpicked them as his followers? That makes them leaders. They've seen all the miracles. They've even healed a few people themselves. What they really want to find out is which *one* of them is the greatest. Each has a mental list of his accomplishments, his achievements, his spiritual résumé. But Jesus's answer stuns them.

"You want to know the truth? You see this little child here?" Jesus reaches over and pulls a small child into their circle. "You want to be the greatest in heaven? Then change your proud heart and make yourself as humble and needy as this little one. Then you are fit for heaven. That's how you become great in my kingdom."

They must have reeled at these words, looked with astonishment at the little boy or girl whom he had pulled into their midst. A barefoot child who did not know his right from his left, a girl with messy hair who could not yet even dress herself, a boy just learning to speak who would starve if not fed by his mother or father.

In my sixth month I did not yet know if I could start over and welcome one more, if I could return to bending and yielding my life to an infant's every need and cry. But I realized that day in the nursery that no one gets promoted above babies and small children. This is part of life—caring for the helpless. We don't get to move on, as though despising weakness. We are to tend the weak and needy always. No one graduates from the call to love and serve.

And when, in that work of pouring our lives into the little ones given to us, we ourselves become like them—dependent, vulnerable, humbled—something great is happening: we are being fit for heaven.

The Third Trimester

Seven

Carrying On

At seven months of pregnancy your baby weighs more
than 2 pounds and looks more like a newborn. His body is
well formed. Fingernails are starting to cover his fingertips.
He can now open and close his eyes
and may turn toward a source of bright light.

—WWW.BABYCENTER.COM

Listen to me, O house of Jacob,
all you who remain of the house of Israel,
you whom I have upheld since you were conceived,
and have carried since your birth....
I am he, I am he who will sustain you.
I have made you and I will carry you.

—ISAIAH 46:3–4

S ome couples plan their pregnancies obsessively, with requests, needs, and preparations listed in detail long before the test stick turns a color. A healthy child first, of course. Choice of gender is usually next. Wishes for color of hair and eyes, who she should look like, whose talents he would inherit. Names are chosen. There are conversations about the ideal spacing between siblings. Arrangements and timetables are set for work and career changes to accommodate a hoped-for child. Plans are made to remodel the guest room into a nursery. A new regimen of exercise and healthy food begins before trying to conceive.

Those of us in this book, and most readers of these pages, didn't get to do any of this—not this time at least. This pregnancy has come in the midst of lives not ready for another life. We are busy, too busy; we are already stretched. We don't have the money, we don't have the energy, maybe we don't have support from our spouse or boyfriend, or maybe there's no one at all to help. While our own bodies create a perfect environment for this new baby, the environment we live in is less than perfect—often far less. Yet we continue. And now it is the seventh month. Our bellies are growing ever larger, the reality of this coming child ever closer. We are beginning to change, to try to ready ourselves for what is coming, but in the meantime we live one day, then the next day. We carry on.

Shoshana had a lot to carry. Her surprise pregnancy came in the midst of a busy life caring for her eldest daughter, in a wheelchair, and her two other daughters. She was angry when she found out, then scared, wondering how she was going to do it all, especially with the needs of her oldest. Before the discovery, two trips had been planned—one to Las Vegas for her best friend's wedding and a family trip to Disney World. Once Shoshana and Jon found out, they decided to keep their travel plans. Though she was eight months pregnant while posing with Mickey Mouse and traipsing the miles of exhibits and rides, it was a good time for their family, and the pregnancy was going much better than the last. They were hopeful, and they knew, happily, that this baby was a boy. Then, in the middle of their vacation, they got a phone call.

It was a friend from back home who served with Jon in the National Guard. "We're going to Iraq," said the voice. "Our unit's been put on alert. I'm not sure when we're going, but it's soon." Jon and Shoshana were stunned. Shoshana could hardly think about it. Here they were in Disney World, a dream-come-true vacation for their family, and it would end like this. *No,* she decided with bulldog determination. *I'm not going to let this news ruin our vacation.* They finished their time there, both Jon and Shoshana focusing on the girls, holding their own worries at bay.

The official word came shortly after they returned home: Jon's National Guard unit was to leave in two weeks for two months of training in Texas. They would return home for Christmas, and then they would be deployed to Iraq for eighteen to twenty-four months.

It happened so fast that Shoshana felt numb. She hardly had time to think about what all this meant. She would deliver this baby alone. She would raise him alone for the next two years. She had three other girls to care for, one with frequent medical emergencies. Jon would have to close down his business, leaving them with very little income.

Two days before Jon left, perhaps registering the shock and stress, Shoshana went into preterm labor. Lying in the hospital, hooked up to monitors, Jon beside her, she realized with almost unbearable sadness and anger that all of this was indeed going to happen. It could have been a joyous time of life: they had adjusted to the surprise entrance of this child, and it was a hoped-for boy. The girls were so excited; their family would be complete. But in the face of Jon's absence, where was the joy? How could she do all this by herself?

Shoshana moved between anger at what was happening to her family and beseeching prayer.

Jon did leave as scheduled that Friday. The contractions that day were stopped with medication, and Shoshana went home to await the final weeks of her pregnancy.

Randi was teaching full-time and had just started a master's program, with classes meeting mostly at night. She knew it was going to be tough to do both, but she was single and had no other commitments. When her period was late two or three weeks, it didn't bother her until, one night, she woke out of a dead sleep with a panicked thought: *What if I'm pregnant!* She hadn't considered it before, because she had slept with this man just once. He was only her second boyfriend, though Randi was in her thirties.

Randi was pregnant, of course. When the home test bloomed pink, her world spun, but not out of control. She knew she would not have an abortion; she had already done that and had vowed never again. Randi had always hoped that someday she might have a child. This was not how or what or when she expected it, but she would not turn this away. What about her graduate program? She forced herself to calmly think it through. Classes ended in March, and her due date was April. Yes, it would work. She would continue.

For the next nine months she taught all day, then on

Tuesdays and Thursdays drove to downtown Chicago for classes that met from six until ten o'clock. On Saturdays the classes met all day. Walking from the parking lot to the campus every class night, Randi would take a few steps, throw up, walk a little farther, then throw up again. It was partly the pregnancy, partly the tremendous stress she felt.

But the load she was carrying soon doubled. Because her belly was growing so fast, her doctor did another ultrasound—she was pregnant with twins. Randi could hardly absorb the news, but because her life felt so empty of love, she believed there would be room for two instead of one. For their sakes now and for her own, she could not give up her employment and this degree that would increase her pay. She would need it now more than ever. As a first-year teacher in a low-paying district, her salary was only nineteen thousand dollars. She was living in a mobile home and paying four hundred dollars a month for rent, leaving her with very little for bills, for baby clothes, for anything other than essentials. She kept going in her job, her degree program, her pregnancy, in spite of twins, in spite of unsympathetic professors who made no allowances for her, in spite of being alone.

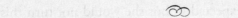

Michele Gonzales went through her surprise pregnancy with four children, living in an eleven-hundred-square-foot apartment on a remote island in the Aleutians in Alaska, where it blew and rained and stormed almost continually. Her husband was busy with work, and Michele stayed at home all day with the kids, homeschooling, fighting off cabin fever and the bickering that intensifies through the long, dark winter. And then the complications and worry about the baby, the long-distance flights for tests and exams.

Teresa Carlson at eight months pregnant was put in a wheelchair because of her swelling, placenta previa, and early contractions. The doctors advised her to leave her rural home and relocate close to the hospital, some 250 miles away. Though they needed her husband's income, Rome would not leave Teresa but left his job instead to make the move with her. With no employment and no income, they struggled to find a place to rent and to scrape together enough money for food and for cab fare for doctor appointments. Finally public assistance came through after weeks of battling red tape and empty cupboards.

My second surprise pregnancy came in the middle of a crisis in our family business and a house-building project gone bad: the walls and roof of our house that fronted the ocean were found to be rotten, requiring new walls, virtually a new house. We had to move out. We packed up the entire household, room by room, to move to a small apartment, a temporary displacement that lasted seven months, four months past the birth of the baby. The four boys slept in the garage. Our finances were ransacked. Our family business in question. Our economic future uncertain.

∞

Each of us wanted calm, an orderly life, an uncomplicated pregnancy. Wasn't it enough that we were making room for another child without all the rest, all the other crises and disruptions? Weren't we giving away enough already? I don't know if anyone can answer the why of this, why some are asked to carry so much. But every woman I know and met kept going, kept getting up in the morning, kept dressing and eating and growing her baby as she walked through each day.

Carrying on is like the paradox of birth itself—the bearing down each day with a ferocity you didn't know you possessed, and with it also the letting go, suspending full knowledge, full sight, full understanding of all that is happening. This is sometimes simply a walk by faith: faith that there is a higher purpose than you can see at the moment, faith that the Maker of all life has not made a mistake, no matter what you're feeling, faith that the One who called you to this work will supply what you need. And it is a walk by knowledge—this even more sure than faith—that in carrying this child you are giving her or him the chance to *be*. Without *being* what else matters?

Do you see the immensity of what you are doing? Carry on.

Eight

Making Changes

Your baby is getting too big to move around much,

but its kicks are stronger, and you may be able to see

the outline of a small heel or elbow against your abdomen.

Your baby is now 16 to 18 inches long

and weighs about four pounds.

—WWW.FOLSOMOBGYN.COM

There is a time for everything,

and a season for every activity under heaven:

a time to be born and a time to die,

a time to plant and a time to uproot…

a time to tear down and a time to build.

—ECCLESIASTES 3:1–3

L ess than eight weeks to go. The countdown begins. At thirty weeks I would change my measuring ritual and now count down instead of up: seven weeks to go, six weeks to go. It collapsed my sense of time, lifted a bit of its weight from me, even as I grew heavier and slower. As birth nears, for many it is the time to make larger shifts, to move from thought to action, sometimes physically pushing aside the things in your life that don't belong with pregnancy or with a newborn infant in the house.

For those of us living out this unplanned pregnancy, the change and upheaval to our lives as the baby approaches is often greater than for those who have waited until their circumstances were just right. Lifestyles may need to change radically and quickly: leaving high school or college; getting a job to support the baby; moving to a new apartment with an extra bedroom; quitting a job and preparing to stay home with the baby; throwing away the cigarettes and wine bottles…

For many women the changes they make to accommodate this new life end up changing the entire direction of their lives.

∽

Dawna was living high and hard. Married at fifteen, divorced soon after. Drinking, doing drugs, supplying cocaine to her friends, working in a bar, no responsibilities. All of it an escape from a family that provided little caring and plenty of abuse and neglect. Dawna grew up fast and was determined that no one would push her around and force her to do anything again. She would do as she pleased.

At twenty she met Dave and fell in love. They planned to marry in three months. Then Dawna turned up pregnant. She cried bitterly, scared that the very thing her great-grandmother had warned against most of her childhood had now happened: she would be tied down by a baby. She had heard those messages all her life: "Babies tie you down. You can't go anywhere, you can't do anything once you've got a baby. They're a lot of trouble." Dawna believed these messages. Now she had lost her freedom, and she and Dave wouldn't have any time alone together. It wasn't the way she wanted to start her marriage. The good life was over.

Once she knew she was pregnant, and the tears finally dried up, Dawna took a hard look at her life and realized she had to make some changes. No more drugs, no more drinking. She was scared to quit it all cold turkey, but she couldn't hurt this baby, who would be hers and Dave's, no matter how she felt about it now. That move alone changed the direction of her life. And then, three years after her daughter was born, she had another daughter.

"Dave rescued me, and my two babies rescued me," Dawna says now. She lists family members and friends who have become prostitutes, who are in jail or on the streets. "I could be on the streets, still drugging. But when I had those babies, they were so dependent on me, I realized I had to provide for them. I had such a drive to provide for them. I'd go to the store, and instead of just buying whatever I wanted, I'd think of them, what was good for them, what they needed. I stopped focusing just on myself. I started to budget and started thinking ahead to the future instead of just right now. When Dave and I would fight, I'd want to leave, but I knew the girls needed us to make a better effort. I took more time to make decisions. Having the girls changed everything. Everything. I don't think there's anything about my life that is the same as it was before I had children. My life was going nowhere."

Lori Harford was sixteen when she became pregnant, seventeen when her daughter was born. Like Dawna, she was running with a party crowd. She had grown up in church and knew better but couldn't seem to stop. "I was hanging out with people who were dragging me down. I was not doing well. I wasn't living the way I should have been, and I knew it."

Lori and her boyfriend, Justin, were deeply shaken over

this pregnancy. She tried to continue going to school—she was a junior, just a year and a half till graduation—but she couldn't focus; she couldn't get rid of the shame or the fear that people would find out. After several weeks of walking from class to class with her head down, bundled in bulky sweaters, Lori just couldn't do it anymore.

She felt like a failure for quitting school, but she and Justin were moving forward. They started going to church together for the first time. They went to counseling, and through the counseling and the knowledge that they had a child coming who would need them both, they deepened their commitment to each other. Two months later they were married.

Now, with her baby fifteen months old, Lori is studying to get her GED and plans to start school in the fall at a community college. Her life has radically changed direction since she first saw those two bold lines on the pregnancy stick.

"If I had continued to live the way I was living, I don't know where I would be now. I look back and see my old friends, what they're doing. Most of them are dropouts. All they're focused on is, When do I get drugs? Who has the cooler friends? I don't know why I glamorized that kind of lifestyle before. It was almost like a blindness. That could still be me.

"Justin has changed a lot too. He's a different person than he was before. He loves his baby so much. He wants to be a dad that she can look up to and admire. I'm very pleased with where I am right now. We're living with my mother, and I still have my struggles and still have a long way to go, but I feel like God rescued me through my daughter. Even though I wasn't doing right, still God used it in my life for good."

Each of the women who said to me, in near whispers, "This baby saved my life," knew she was making new choices that would move her toward life and light, away from addictions and destruction. Yes, they were giving up, but the gains were so much greater that the choice was clear.

Sometimes making lesser changes can feel harder. Giving up professions and career paths can feel like giving up parts of our very selves.

Theresa Peterson had fished commercially in the cold Alaskan waters most of her adult life and had managed to fit a fishing schedule around the mothering of her two children. She loved working out on the ocean, the freedom and independence it gave her, the income from one or two months' work that saved her from having to work the rest of the year so she could focus entirely on her husband and children. When she turned up pregnant at forty, she agonized over losing this one part of her life that had remained a constant. At nearly five months pregnant and already committed to making this one-month halibut trip, Theresa kept her plans and went out as always. Though the trip was taxing and pushed her to her limits, she was not ready to give it up. She still hoped to find a way to accommodate both a baby and one spring fishing trip each year. But then she thought out the details, like keeping up her milk supply while being gone for that month. Theresa tried to envision herself pumping milk on the boat while at sea. This was a hard image to call to mind. Where would she do it? There was only one place for privacy—a bathroom so small you could hardly even turn around. Several times a day she'd have to stop work, come down from the deck, take off her rain gear, sit there on the toilet seat—pump to breast—while everyone compensated for her absence up on deck.

Theresa remembers that time. "I wanted to do it all. I wanted my own taste of independence and freedom, which is what fishing is for me. It was such an important part of my life for so long that it was hard to let it go."

But she did. She hasn't been out on a fishing trip for three years. Yet two years after her daughter was born, it was her fishing experience that landed her a prize job as a coordinator for a marine conservation group. "I never expected to have a job like this. I really like it. It's a whole new direction for me, but it's exciting."

Donna, a self-described workaholic who loved her job as receptionist and bookkeeper for a dentist, cut back to half time when her surprise child was born. "Jacob's arrival really changed how I viewed my work. I felt like I gained a completely different perspective."

Bianca Clark, during her pregnancy, left her college musical theater program that she had worked so hard to enter. She knew she would have to work to support her new family and that her attention would be torn between her studies and her daughter. She hopes to return to school in the future. Until then, she is working three jobs and saving her money. "It's not exactly the plan I had, but maybe that wasn't the right plan. This is a new life we've created. Just because it's not the same path I decided on before doesn't mean that I'm a failure, that I can't go back to school. The first time this baby smiles at me I know it will be worth all I've given up."

For me, after discovering the second unplanned pregnancy, I decided I would give up my academic career for good. I would hand it over, walk away from what I had thought I wanted and worked toward for twenty years. Four years of college, five years of graduate school, a résumé that had grown to five pages, and finally the job I wanted: a tenure-track position as assistant professor of English at a state university.

After five years in the job, I sat on a plane on my way to an academic conference. No one at the college knew yet that I was pregnant or that I would soon be resigning because of it. I was acutely aware that this was my last flight as an English professor. I sat against the window, dressed in a roomy black wool jumper, a black trench coat, and black leather shoes. The flight was an hour, time enough to get some classwork done. I pulled out my laptop and began to type.

As I worked, I overheard laughter. Across the aisle, two women sat together, both overweight, dressed in jeans, sneakers, and sport jackets. They were good friends obviously and, I soon learned, both mothers of small children. They were discussing their toddlers' toilet-training experiences in voices loud enough for the front half of the plane to hear.

"When did you start training Christopher?"

"Much too soon! He wasn't ready. I could never get him to put his penis down—he calls it a pee-pee—and he'd end up spraying all over the bathroom walls!"

The other woman hooted and began her own urine-in-the-wrong-places story. And soon they graduated to narratives of poop.

I was listening to this, of course. I couldn't help it. I almost smiled at the irony of it, knowing the visible contrasts between us: I was the one in heels, working a laptop, on deadline, flying alone, obviously on business, yet I had five children at home, one slightly more than a year old. And another on the way. I could tell my own potty-training combat stories. *But I don't. And I don't do it in public,* I thought, feeling disdain for these housewives. My stomach twisted at this visible reminder of where I was headed again. I thought of all I was letting go of, that soon I would be like them, flying in sneakers and jeans, talking about my kids' excrement or, worse, cleaning it up. And not caring who knew about it.

And then, sometime during that trip, I heard myself. Who did I think I was? I still had so far to go.

In my eighth month of pregnancy, I was back in the same city, with Abraham now, almost two years old, and Duncan, who was there on business. I was no longer an English professor. Though I was there to give a writing workshop at the university and was working on this book, I was mostly stay-at-home, pregnant-mom Leslie, just trying to get through the pregnancy and trying to keep the rest of my family in the essentials.

While waiting for Duncan's meeting to finish on a Sunday afternoon, I stayed with Abraham in the foyer of a corporate office building. We waited for more than thirty minutes, during which time I attempted to contain Abraham's destruction of the water cooler, the neat stack of paper cups, the carpet, my clothes. He got me partly wet; I was tired, on my knees picking up cups, my body overwhelmed with a load I could hardly carry. Then the elevator bell rang.

Out stepped a woman dressed in an impeccable black wool suit, black hose, spike heels, with an elegant strand of pearls around her neck, her hair stylish, her makeup extensive. She was calm, professional, and in full control. I was none of these things. And I knew her. I had interviewed her for a book I had written years earlier.

"Oh! Leslie! How are you?" she queried as she glanced quickly at my belly, her face trying to hide the obvious astonishment. We were close to the same age.

"I'm doing well," I fibbed, equally shocked at her appearance. Why did she look as if she were about to attend the opera rather than a casual weekend meeting in a closed-down building where everyone else was wearing jeans?

We struggled to make small talk to cover our mutual discomfort while I tried to keep Abraham in line, and then she walked coolly down the hall to her meeting. I knew what I looked like in her eyes: the eternally pregnant woman with no political or social influence, a woman of the house. A loser in the Mommy wars. Her children were nearly grown and gone. But I felt no envy for her. I didn't need to be there anymore. I knew what that was like; I knew her sense of self and significance was based mostly on how others viewed her. I had lived in both places, and one was not higher than the other. One was harder; there was no question. I had been called back to the harder work.

Maybe I was almost ready then. I knew the changes I had made in my life were right and good: I was leaving the work I loved for the work of loving another.

We all do it, make changes as we wait for the birth of our baby, make room in our lives, our houses, our work, our hearts. Changes that feel hard at the time, that *are* hard at the time. But we do it anyway, believing that something of greater value is coming.

Nine

Birth

The baby is now about eight times bigger than it was at
three months…and has increased in weight approximately
600 times. Most of the lanugo has dropped off.…
The fingernails extend beyond the fingers
and may need cutting at birth.

—*THE COMPLETE BOOK OF PREGNANCY
AND CHILDBIRTH*

Whoever welcomes a little child
like this in my name welcomes me.

—MATTHEW 18:5

I t is almost time. Never has time moved so slowly as in these last two weeks. You know the baby can come at any moment. You are living in a kind of slow-motion suspension, your very molecules weighted with lead. The list of complaints is long:

"This is it! I'm about to abandon this ridiculous body! Someone get me out of here!"

"I just want to be able to sleep at night. That's all. To just change positions without having to heave and grunt and wake my husband up. I can't wait!"

"I've been sleeping on the floor on one air mattress on top of another—I feel like the princess and the pea, and I'm still never comfortable."

"I've been stuffed up and congested this whole last month. I can't wait to breathe properly."

"I'm tired of everyone asking me, 'Haven't you had that baby yet?' "

"I'm so big and uncomfortable that an old guy at my church told me it hurt him just looking at me."

But something has happened over all these weeks that you didn't expect. You are ready for this baby. Or, at the least, you are ready *not* to be pregnant. The space the two of you are sharing within a single stretch of skin will burst, you think. You feel like a whale with Jonah inside. A bus with too many passengers. You cannot wait to have your own body back, to roll over in bed anytime you want, to breathe easily, to climb the stairs without gripping the rail, to put on your old jeans, to walk lightly... All this is coming.

You're tired, too, of carrying all the what-if's: the anxieties, the uncertainties, the doubts. You've run through the worst-case scenarios so many times that the scenes roll at the touch of a button. You're ready to live out what comes rather than what might be.

All the discomforts of these last weeks—nausea, Braxton Hicks contractions, sleeplessness, maybe even false labor— are readying you as well, preparing your body for this final push. And they have readied your mind. The coming labor and birth that were the focus of so much apprehension and dread through these months, now you welcome. The fiery trial of birth will be the moment of release for you and for this baby. Bring it on.

∞

What happens in those moments and hours of birth can be transformational. Nearly every movie that includes a birth shows an exhausted but elated woman lying, receiving the just-born infant into her arms, her face glowing, the husband or partner on fire in love as he cuddles both his woman and his child. In cynical moments it is easy to wonder if Hollywood is just running commercials for Hallmark cards. If this is your first birth, you wonder, how can it be *that* miraculous, *that* magical, *that* different from the rest of life? And is it really possible to love a creature you've only just met who doesn't even look quite finished? But I am here, along with others, to say, "Yes, this really happens. Birth can be the highest, most amazing moment of your life. It feels like nothing less than a miracle."

For Pam Tripp it was miraculous. This was the pregnancy she didn't want—another pregnancy meant another miscarriage. She had had too many already since her only child had been born ten years earlier. Pam held her emotions in check throughout the months, fearing another loss. The day for the scheduled C-section finally came. It all felt surreal to her— the hospital gown, the nurses. The last time she had been in the hospital and had been prepped for surgery was after a miscarriage. Though her husband and daughter were spilling over with excitement, Pam's emotions were numb—would it all go well? The baby was not in her arms yet.

Soon her body was numb as well, as the doctors partially sedated her and then gave her a spinal block. When it had taken full effect, the doctor made the incision—Pam felt nothing. But as they scooped and lifted the baby head-first from her womb, with the baby's legs and torso still deep in her body, Sarah Elisabeth announced her presence and began crying the high-pitched, urgent cry of the just born. Pam was shocked fully awake by this sound—this baby, breathing her first air, crying her first cry, *was still inside her!*

Later, when the nurses brought the cleaned and tightly wrapped newborn back to Pam's room and placed her in her arms, Pam, not given to emotional displays, sobbed. This pregnancy she didn't want, this child she never expected was now here, and Pam could only weep. In front of her parents, her husband, her daughter, the nurses, she was overcome with a sense of completion. As Sarah made her way to Pam's breast and latched on with a never-let-go strength, Pam stopped crying. There was no need to cry anymore. Everything was as it should be.

Theresa Peterson's whole family—her husband and two older children—were there by her bed as she labored. When

Elizabeth entered the world, Theresa's son and daughter were scared by their mother's pain but wide eyed at their new little sister. They adored the baby instantly and held and cuddled her as if they knew just what to do. It was a changing point for the whole family. Theresa realized this wasn't just about her having a baby—her entire family was gaining someone else to love. This baby became the burning light of their house.

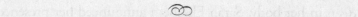

The experience of birth is the highlight of many women's lives. But it's important to know these emotions aren't experienced by everyone. For some, the moment of birth does not bring revelation and immediate joy.

Jill Rohrer lay on the table in the labor room in the throes of labor pains. She was scared—she had never done this before. She had been pregnant for nine months, so she knew something about pregnancy but nothing about birth, and here it was, upon her in such force. And the father of this baby, whom she had once hoped to marry, was gone and was never coming back. She ached with loneliness. The contractions seemed to keep pace with these emotions, pulling harder and longer. The nurses encouraged her, "You're going to have this baby soon! The baby is coming soon—hang in there!" After a particularly hard contraction, Jill retorted, "Stop telling me I'm having a baby! Stop telling me the baby will be here soon! I don't want to hear that I'm having a baby!" That was still the very thing she feared.

Jill had worked right up until the birth; her first teaching job and staying healthy on her feet consumed her every moment. She hadn't thought concretely yet about another person coming. And here this person was, just about to emerge. *I'm not ready,* Jill thought. *How can I do this?* She had been having dreams—ridiculous dreams—that she had given birth to a cat. *Oh! A cat!* She had thought, *How simple! I can take care of a cat!* But this was no dream.

After a long labor, it finally ended, and a baby girl was placed in her arms. Jill felt as though she were in shock. She looked down at this infant and knew in the back of her mind that she was supposed to feel love, that this was supposed to be *the* moment, but it wasn't. She couldn't muster up any feelings except loneliness and fatigue and an immense responsibility as the only parent of this child.

Shoshana was in and out of the hospital throughout her last two months. Contractions would come and would intensify until they were three to five minutes apart, and Shoshana would drive to the hospital, sure each time this was it. On this day, November 11, the contractions came again, harder now. This time the date was right. At the hospital the nurse was ready to send her home again—she was still dilated to three centimeters, as she had been for weeks—but suddenly everything began to happen very fast. Within an hour and a half the baby was born.

Shoshana lay back, wrung out by the intensity of the birth. Just five seconds later, three deep breaths later, the nurse handed her new son, Jayson, to her. She filled her eyes with his tiny body: he was perfectly formed, with dark hair, dark blue eyes, long thin fingers. As she held him, Shoshana felt exhausted and empty. This moment should have been so other than it was. She knew her husband would be with her if he weren't overseas, but it wasn't right, just her and the baby. She felt overwhelmingly sad.

Lori Harford, seventeen, was afraid to look at her daughter when the nurse brought her to her bed. This was the moment of truth. Had she done everything right during the pregnancy? Would it be her fault if something was wrong? Though Justin and she had married, and though their lives had turned around completely because of this coming child, there was still guilt and doubt. Would she truly be able to love and care for this baby when she was little more than a child herself? As Kariona was placed in her arms, Lori wanted to love her baby instantly—she had heard other women speak of this—but she was so tired, and there were so many other questions. How could she finish high school? Would Justin make enough to support them all? Would they ever have a place of their own? How could she mother a child when she still needed her own mother? Her new baby, though tiny, felt heavy in her arms.

⌒

I knew about head-over-heels falling in love with a being just minutes old. The narrative of my first four births would read like a mushy romance of amazing loves and emotional highs that can hardly be held down with words. But with my two surprise children, how could I possibly feel this same exhilaration after pregnancies mired in doubt, relinquishment, and conflict? The sixth pregnancy in particular had been almost more than I could bear. What now would come at this birth?

The answer was given on November 23, a day that was significant for more than one reason. When I first discovered this last pregnancy, the due date given was November 18. I remember feeling irritated that it was so close to my birthday. Prayers throughout the pregnancy grew more urgent as the time grew close: "Lord, I have given up so much already. Surely you won't take my birthday from me too?"

The day began with contractions early in the morning. By five o'clock I was at the hospital, strapped to monitors, watching the needle climb successions of squiggly mountains as the pain cinched my belly. I knew this was the day of birth. It was just as I feared; my birthday would now always be *his* birthday. Between contractions, catching my breath, I thought about the statistics. What were the chances of birthing five boys in a row? Or having two unplanned pregnancies in a row in your forties? And out of 365 possible days of birth, what were the chances that he would be born precisely on this one day I wanted to keep for myself?

By this point I was no longer angry. It was all so designed, so statistically unlikely, as against all odds as his conception, that I could only surrender. My birthday was the one last thing I was holding on to, and now that was gone, taken. The final erasure of self. I had nothing else to give, it felt, though that was far from true. And I was astounded. How did God know that it would take all this for me to believe? That it would take all this for me to know that this new son was not an accident, not a mistake, not an afterthought? That he was a surprise only to me? Nothing about him was a surprise to God.

There were mercies this day. Among them, that the labor was the quickest and least painful of all my births. That Duncan and my sister-in-law Beth were there. That I didn't tear or bleed excessively.

When Micah was placed on my chest, straight from my womb, I do not know exactly what I felt, but the moment is contained in a photo taken by my sister-in-law: a ghostly white baby, plump, lies vertical in the bed of the doctor's hands. It is just a single second or two since he slipped out of me, was caught, held, and lifted to me. My face still registers the shock of release, the sudden cessation of pain, the first gasp of air I am breathing for myself alone. And in that same breath, he is there, one arm raised, fingers open close to my face, reaching for me. I almost didn't see this greeting; it happened so quickly. I just knew he was here, he was my son, he needed me, and I would receive him.

∞

Your baby is in your arms now. She has come already knowing the pitch of your voice, the smell of your milk, the cadence of your sentences, the rhythm of your walk. She has arrived loving you. With all the needs of her being, with all of her senses, with everything she has, she loves you—because *you have given her life*. You *are* her life.

Maybe, though, you are holding your newborn knowing he will soon be placed into others' arms. You have carried this child for nine months; you have birthed him. Do you love this baby now? How can you love what you are letting go? But love is much more than what you feel; it is above all, what you do. You may be creating a family for a couple who could not have one otherwise. You are creating a future for your son or daughter that you know you could not give by yourself. You are doing something very hard *because* of your love for this child.

If you are bringing your baby home with you, these moments just after birth are your first chance to welcome your baby. But you may feel nothing right now other than an overpowering fatigue—as indeed you should. You have just accomplished the hardest, the greatest, the most essential feat the human being is capable of. Hold your baby for as long or as little as you need in these first minutes, then sleep. Don't worry; it is only your first chance, not your last. There are so many chances ahead, so many more welcomes for your son or daughter. Every morning, every moment, another chance. I know—we want a flood, a sudden up-welling of emotions and tenderness that sweeps us away into the land of love, baby in arms. But the waters can trickle too, gathering slowly, rising over the days and weeks into something you begin to name as love. It will keep rising, the waters deepening over the months, until you know for certain this *is* love, a deeper love than you have ever known before. It came to every woman in this book. It will surely come to you.

For now, in whatever time you are given, rest, knowing you are a woman of strength and courage. Every woman who brings forth a child can be called the same, but you have done more. You did not give in to fear. You did not listen to those who may have urged you to end this pregnancy. You have changed your life, sustained other losses to bring this baby to light and air. And now you have something to show for those months and sacrifices: beautiful bone and flesh and blood of your very bone. But there is more. You are more than who you once were. You emerge from this birth more resilient and resourceful, wiser and deeper than the woman who stared unbelieving at a test stick forty weeks ago. You have traveled so far and done so much. Rest now in all you have created and become.

Epilogue

After Birth

While you were pregnant, your body worked
round-the-clock for forty weeks to help your baby grow.
Now that your baby is here, there's more work to be done
as your body recovers from pregnancy, labor, and delivery.

—*PLANNING YOUR PREGNANCY AND BIRTH*

Bring my sons from afar
and my daughters from the ends of the earth—
everyone who is called by my name,
whom I created for my glory,
whom I formed and made.

—ISAIAH 43:6–7

The pregnancy is over! Your body is not quite your own yet—you still do not recognize it. Your breasts are full of milk and now belong to someone else. As does your schedule. You will need to heal from tearing or an episiotomy or a C-section.

But everything feels different. A new story begins. This beginning is so much more tangible than the other. The other beginning was real too: the conception, the month-by-month growth of the baby within you, the incredible experience of birth. But you know now as you hold your baby that all this was a warmup, an introduction, and now you are living the full story.

This beginning will not be easy or simple. Perhaps it may even feel like the hardest part of all with nightly interruptions, loss of sleep, constant feedings, the moment-by-moment reality of caring for a newborn. But every week that goes by gets perceptively better, every month easier. As someone who has lived this out six times, I can tell you it is not just a cliché—it is true.

∞

What is possible for you and your baby now? Anything. I know this because of my own life and because of the women I have watched and listened to these past four years who are living and growing and thriving since the birth of their unplanned babies. Even those who resisted the pregnancy the most. In these final words, I want you to hear where some of these women are now and who these unplanned pregnancies have become.

Lori Harford's daughter, Kariona, is now eighteen months old, with black hair and striking blue eyes. Lori is relishing her every achievement, her first giggle at three months, her first reach for a toy, her first spoken word. "Every new little thing that she does makes my heart sing. Nobody has that joy for their child but the mother and father." She is astounded at the changes in herself since the baby was born. "I have a friend who told me about her abortion. She said she thought she was too selfish to buy things for the baby instead of things for herself, so she knew she wasn't ready to have a baby. I used to think I would be the same way, but everything changes once you see your baby. Now I buy clothes to make her look cute, and it doesn't matter so much about me. It all changes."

Jill Rohrer is no longer a working single parent; four years after Ashley's birth, she married Dan. Ashley is now an energetic and independent eight-year-old in third grade and is the proud big sister to Emily and Mary.

"Ashley has brought so much to my life that I didn't

expect. She's brought an awareness of how awfully selfish I can be and how selfless I can be. There are times when I would do anything for her but other times when what she needs or wants is the last thing on my mind. Through her, I've learned that love is both a chosen commitment and a feeling and that the choice remains constant as the feelings ebb and flow around it. I am so humbled and so honored that God placed her in my care here on earth."

Michael Schwarz's surprise pregnancy meant she would have three children three years old and under. It was one of the hardest times in her life. Her daughter, Rebeckah, is now two and a half years old.

"God knew what he was doing when I had Becca. We have a special bond because of all we've gone through, the whole process of my thinking I didn't want her. I look at her, and I see myself. She has my personality—the feistiness at times and then the tender spirit. Even her looks. I look at her and see me. There's something about her eyes. There's something very special that God did to this little girl to grab me in the gut. I'll always have this bond with her. I wouldn't ever trade her."

Shoshana still has more than a year and a half to go raising four children alone, with her husband deployed in Iraq. Jayson is colicky; Shoshana is exhausted. "I'm nurturing this baby, but the opportunity to really bond has been hard. So much has happened: my husband leaving, the other children, the lack of sleep, the neediness. He's five weeks old now, and it has finally sunk in how devastating it would be if something should happen to him. I'm hanging on by a thread, emotionally, mentally, physically. I just bear down, keep going, push forward. But I've started clinging to Jayson for my strength. I have something so precious in him; I know I'll get through it."

Trisha Pruitt's daughter, Katrina, now three, continues to bring joy to Trisha's life. "I had lost my own identity in a house of all boys. Katrina has been an answer to prayer. I feel like I found myself again through her, that it's okay to be female, it's okay to cry, it's okay to be upset. She's brought such a softness in the house. The boys are learning how to handle girls better. Now that I'm farther down the line, I can say that I'm really glad we ended up having another baby, though it was hard at first. Now Steve and I feel complete."

Marianne's baby survived the abortion her mother forced her to have at age sixteen. To support herself and her new daughter, Laurel, Marianne at age eighteen began a small business out of her family's home. After several years she expanded to a larger store as her business grew. Laurel recently graduated with top honors from a prestigious university. She makes her home between two countries, the Dominican Republic and the United States, and is soon to be married. Marianne says of Laurel, "I'm very proud of all that she has done and who she is. I'm so happy with her."

Marianne later married and is now raising two children and running a successful business with her husband.

Michele Gonzales's son Levi is four years old now. "I'm glad that it happened. I'm thrilled we have him. After not wanting another baby, then having another, it turned out to be an unexpected treat that I got to do all those things over again, for the last time, knowing it was the last time. And having him force us to settle down, to quit moving around so much, which has been good. Levi's not an angel. He can be a real stinker. I think everybody has spoiled him. But of all my kids right now, he's the one who loves me the most. He's the one who has to run to the door to kiss me good-bye. He wants to go with me wherever I'm going. He's my little companion."

Randi's twin sons are now fifteen, sophomores in high school. She has raised them alone, supporting them through full-time teaching; she never married. "I never felt sorry for myself or desperate or alone in their younger years. I felt capable of taking care of them. Their dependence on me never scared me. They gave me a reason to live. I wasn't lonely anymore.

"In these teen years, though, it has gotten harder. I have never regretted having them, but I have regretted having them without a husband. The older they get, the more they want a father. It's been a very big struggle for me. But on the other hand, I know they are a gift from God. I knew that the minute I found out I was pregnant. I almost feel as though God looked down and had pity on me. I believe he knew I could live my whole life without a husband, but he knew how badly I wanted a kid. And I got two."

And what of **Linda Ross,** pregnant from rape, who birthed the baby, then relinquished her to an adoption agency? How does this story, begun in such pain, end? Thirty years after she signed the papers, when her own three children with her husband, Alan, had grown and left the house, Linda began a search for her daughter. The search didn't take long; mother and daughter were reunited soon after Linda started looking for her.

"Saturday morning my family and I went to pick up Stacey and her husband. I was a basket case. I was just weeping. I could not stop! We went through the airport. As I got out of the car, I was weeping; as I went in, I was weeping. And then she came through the gate. I knew her immediately. It was about two minutes of awkwardness, and that was it. She was crying as I was weeping, holding her; then we introduced her to everyone, and we just stood there together for a minute. The reality of this, actually seeing her and touching her and holding her was unbelievable, just a sense of wholeness again and of belonging.

"I keep coming back to those verses in Psalm 126 that I had marked and dated the night before she was born: 'Those who sow in tears will reap with songs of joy. He who goes out weeping, carrying seed to sow, will return with songs of joy.' When I think about it still, I am just totally taken that God arranged it all and brought it all to pass in his time. He has brought beauty out of ashes. I look back to the rape and the abuse and all that happened, and I think, like Joseph in the Old Testament, that maybe men meant it for evil, but God meant it for good. He has brought good out of it."

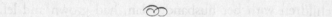

For me, it has been and continues to be a hard journey; I will not lie to you. But so much has happened that I didn't expect since the births of my last sons. I have been pushed beyond my limits often, but my limits and abilities have expanded. My career has taken a better turn and is growing. My other children have learned tenderness and a new kind of love. And my surprise children—they continue to surprise me. Abraham, at three years old, was crying inconsolably. Micah, at nineteen months, toddled over and offered a handful of mashed bananas to Abraham. Abraham took the proffered bananas, swallowed his cries, and cinched his tiny brother in a chest hug. Last week Micah, now nearly two, all twenty-five pounds of him, rushed to his fragile eighty-eight-year-old grandpa's side as DeWitt stood with his cane to walk. Micah's tiny hand reached up to grasp his grandpa's, and with a face of knowing patience and utter concentration, he walked his grandfather slowly to the door.

These are not just moments. My entire life is suffused with the changes and wonders these boys have brought. I am surprised because I did not expect any of this. I am surprised as I watch them grow and become people utterly distinct from my other children, human beings completely themselves: Abraham the tender hearted, who serenades me every day with flowers and happy songs; Micah the lionhearted, who is equally fierce in love and war.

All of us are here in this book to say, yes, the tunnel winds and twists, but it does open into light. It *is* possible to find and make joy. And perhaps it is sweeter because we didn't expect it. We didn't expect to love this unexpected baby as much as we do. We didn't expect her or him to love us as each does. We may have known all about the work, about all the disruption to our lives, but we forgot about the love—his baby cheek against ours, his face buried in our breast as he feeds, his first calls to us alone.

Even more than this, I marvel at the power and force of every single life. All of us could have ended these lives in a few moments, secretly, with only a doctor knowing. We could have gone on with our lives just as planned, trying to maintain control over our bodies and our futures. But who can count or measure what we would have lost? Sometimes as I watch Abraham and Micah, I try to calculate this. I would have lost all that these children are now and are becoming, the huge space that they already fill in this world. I would have lost the parts of myself that are stronger. My children would have lost the adoring company of their young brothers. And what would replace all of this absence and loss? Only a painful lifelong imagining of who they might have been. Now, instead of wondering who they might have become, I wonder at all they are. The surprise continues.

Acknowledgments

Behind every book is a story of Becoming as wondrous and painful, as full of the mysteries of Providence and the labors of the flesh as the creation of every child. This page is an abbreviation of the most important part of this story, which begins with all the women—nearly forty of them—who trusted me with their own stories of unexpected pregnancy. Some let me into their homes while they were still in pajamas, nursing their newborn; some opened their doors and their lives to a complete stranger. Some spoke of feelings and hurts never before revealed. All knew how alone they felt through their pregnancy and welcomed an opportunity to be part of breaking the lonely quiet for others. I could not have written this book without them.

Others who played a major role:

Luci Shaw, whose work and life I have long admired, graciously spoke the right words at the right time. Thank you for every encouragement.

Elisa Stanford, my esteemed editor and new friend, believed in the book from the start and patiently breathed these words to life. This book is yours as well.

The staff and editors at WaterBrook Press, who work cheerfully and diligently, laboring for something lasting. Thank you for hearing us and letting us speak.

Readers' Guide for Individuals or Groups

These questions are provided to help stimulate thought and discussion about your own journey through unexpected pregnancy. They may be used in a group that meets weekly or monthly, perhaps at a pregnancy center, a home, or a church. If such a group doesn't yet exist, consider starting one. All you need to begin is this book and the reader's guide as a starting point for discussion. Your group will know what to do next.

This guide may also be used individually by each reader as she finds a few quiet moments somewhere in her day. By working through the questions, answering as honestly as possible, your path may open before you clearer, perhaps even straighter. This is my hope for you.

Chapter One: The Test

1. When did you first suspect you were pregnant?
2. How was your pregnancy confirmed?
3. What were your first thoughts and fears?
4. You may have strong feelings of anger, blame, or guilt right now. For most women, this is the hardest time of all. Don't try to deal with this alone. Find someone who will understand these feelings and allow you to express them. If you can, find someone who will pray with you and for you. Whatever emotional state you are in right now, there is hope to be found along the way. If you are unsure of what to do, please turn to the Further Resources at the back of this book for additional help.

Chapter Two: Telling

1. Have you told the people who need to know about this pregnancy? If not, what are the difficulties? If you've told the baby's father, did he react the way you expected? How did you want him to react?
2. If you've already broken the news that you're pregnant, how did people react? How did you feel about their reactions?
3. Why do you think your family and others might have reacted the way they did? What would their perspective be?

4. People will ask and comment (sometimes rudely) on your pregnancy as you begin to show. What are some of the comments and questions you have heard so far? Practice responding to people about your pregnancy in an honest but polite way. Write down a few phrases and sentences that you might use.

5. Make a list of the key people you know who strongly support your decision to keep the baby or to entrust the baby to an adoptive family. Ask them if you may call them when you need encouragement and help. If you don't know anyone who can support you, turn to the resources pages at the back of the book for a place to start. There are many people who don't know about you yet who want to help you.

Chapter Three: Heartbeat

1. Have you heard your baby's heartbeat yet?
   a. If yes, how many weeks did you have to wait before you heard it? Describe that time of waiting.
   b. If no, how many more weeks do you need to wait until you hear it? Describe what it feels like right now to be waiting.

2. What was it like when you heard the heartbeat for the first time? Did it change the way you felt about this pregnancy? Did it change the way you felt about your body?

3. Once the heartbeat is heard, the chances for a miscarriage fall dramatically. How do you feel about this?

Chapter Four: Showing

1. Your body and your baby are growing every day. How are you adjusting to your changing shape?

2. What are some of your fears about pregnancy and your body shape?

3. Look back through the chapter and make a list of the different strategies the women used to look and feel better about their bodies. Which strategies could you implement? What are some other things you might do to adjust to and appreciate your changing shape?

4. Talk to several mothers you admire about their pregnancies. Ask them what they did during the pregnancy and afterward to keep themselves healthy and positive.

Chapter Five: Finding Out

1. What kind of tests have you had during this pregnancy? Talk with someone you trust about your decisions on how many and which tests to have done.

2. If you have had an ultrasound or an amniocentesis, what was it like to find out more details about the baby?

3. What surprised you most about seeing and hearing your baby?

4. If you have learned the gender of your child, how has that affected the way you feel about this pregnancy? If you feel disappointed at first, that's okay. That's a good reason for knowing now, so you can adjust and be ready for your son or daughter. There are always advantages to either gender: your daughter gets a brother; your mother gets a granddaughter; your husband gets a son… There *is* good in this. Often you will discover the benefits later, if not now.

5. If you have learned of a potential health problem, seek out someone to talk with and pray with. Any mother who has a baby with health problems grieves the loss of the healthy baby she'd expected. She may also have times of resenting the coming baby because of the depth of that child's needs. Since your child is unexpected, your grief and resentment may be even greater than most. Be aware of this and find someone who will let you express your emotions in all their intensity when you need to.

Chapter Six: Starting Over

1. This chapter talks about life as a graph moving in one direction—your plans for the future. Where were you in your life graph before you found out you were pregnant?

2. If you have other children, what part of starting over feels the hardest to you? Is there something you feel

you missed out on with your other child/children that perhaps this time you could do differently (e.g., nurse longer, work less, hire more childcare, hire less child-care, worry less)?

3. Our culture defines success mostly in terms of money, power, and independence. What other measures of success do you think are more important?

4. Are you as successful in these ways right now as you want to be? How could you be more successful as you move through this pregnancy toward birthing and raising a child?

Chapter Seven: Carrying On

1. It is quite likely that as your pregnancy nears its end, others have been watching and admiring you for car-rying on despite less-than-ideal circumstances. What are some of the difficulties you've had to face in your pregnancy?

2. What are some of the qualities about you that people would notice and admire?

3. What resources and strategies have you relied on to get you this far?

4. What other resources and strategies do you need now as you approach birth? Make a list of all that you feel you need in terms of supplies (diapers, baby clothes) and emotional support. If you don't have a plan for labor and birth yet, check the books

and resources listed at the back of this book to help you prepare. Also, be sure you have at least one person—preferably two people—on call who will commit to being with you through labor and birth.

Chapter Eight: Making Changes

1. Making changes in life is never easy. It can feel harder when you're in a stressful pregnancy. Yet the pregnancy can help you make decisions and act on them quickly. A deadline is coming soon, and a new life depends on your choices. In a few sentences, describe out loud or on paper the kind of mother you want to be to your coming son or daughter.

2. What kind of changes in your life do you sense you might need to make to be that kind of mother? Make a list if that is helpful.

3. Which changes can you make on your own, and which do you need help with?

4. Talk to a knowledgeable friend about the next step— maybe a counselor, a pastor, or a pregnancy-center volunteer.

Chapter Nine: Birth

1. If you have already had your baby, congratulations on your amazing accomplishment! What was your birth experience like?

a. What were you unprepared for? How was it different than you expected?

b. Is your baby who you expected him or her to be?

c. If you held your baby in your arms, did you feel love for him or her right away, as Pam did, or did you feel more like Lori and Jill? Explain.

d. If you have chosen to keep your baby, your new life as the mother of this child has just begun. What do you want to do differently in this new life than you've done before? Write down your intentions and desires on a special piece of paper to keep as a reminder of who you want to be as you begin to raise this child.

2. If you haven't had your baby yet, what are some of your worries as you think about the birth? Are you able to talk with your partner about your fears? How does he feel about the upcoming birth?

3. Talk to one or more mothers you admire about their birth experiences. Share your concerns with them.

Readers' Guide
for Couples

These questions are provided to help you and your partner find ways to talk to each other about your unexpected pregnancy. This is a difficult time for both of you. By working through these questions together, respecting each other's responses even when they are very different from your own, you will gain a deeper understanding of each other. The best gift you can give this coming child is your unity.

Chapter One: The Test

1. This is the hardest time for most couples: fearing an unexpected pregnancy in the middle of your lives, then confirming it. Once the pregnancy was confirmed, you may have had very different responses.

What were your individual thoughts and fears? Explain to your partner how you felt and why you reacted as you did.

2. It's natural at this point to feel guilt or blame for the pregnancy. While it is possible to assign guilt ("You didn't keep track of your cycle"; "You delayed the vasectomy"), the reality is that two of you made this baby. Feelings of guilt will only sap your energy and your hope, and the blame game will only erode the unity you will need to make this pregnancy as successful as possible. What words would you use to describe what you are feeling and thinking about the pregnancy right now? Use this list as a starting point:

Angry	Fearful
Guilty	Overwhelmed
Disappointed	Frustrated
Hopeful	Happy
Discouraged	Defensive
Confused	Lonely

3. You have many weeks ahead to deal with this unexpected event in your lives. Forty weeks of pregnancy will give you time to make the shift from what you had planned for your lives to this new plan. Think of other couples (whether you know them or just know about them) who dealt positively with sudden changes to their lives. How did they grow personally and as a couple through those experiences?

Chapter Two: Telling

1. What has been your strategy for telling others about your pregnancy?

2. How have people reacted to you (both individually and as a couple) when you've told them your news? You probably encountered some hurtful and disappointing responses. Talk about some of these reactions together. Why do you think those people reacted the way they did? What would their perspective be?

3. Practice responding to people about your pregnancy in an honest but polite way. Write down a few phrases and sentences you might use.

4. Name one or more people you know who strongly support your decision either to keep the baby or to entrust the baby to an adoptive family. Ask them if you may call them when you need encouragement and help. If you don't know anyone who can support you, turn to the resources pages at the back of the book and begin there. There are many people who don't know about you yet who want to help you.

Chapter Three: Heartbeat

1. Have you heard your baby's heartbeat yet?
   a. If yes, how many weeks did you have to wait before you heard it? What was that waiting period like for each of you?

    b. If no, how many more weeks do you need to wait until you hear it? Describe what it feels like right now to be waiting.

2. What was it like when you heard the heartbeat for the first time? (If your partner was not able to be there with you during this checkup, try to help him understand this experience.) Did it change the way you felt about this pregnancy? Did it change the way you felt about your body?

3. Once the heartbeat is heard, the chances for a miscarriage fall dramatically. How do you both feel about this?

Chapter Four: Showing

1. Your body and your baby are growing and expanding every day. Women need a lot of support and reassurance that they are still attractive—that this isn't about getting fat but about growing a child. What kind of support do you (the woman) need to have from your partner on this issue?

2. Look back through the chapter and make a list of the different strategies the women in these pages used to look and feel better about their bodies. Which strategies could you implement? What are some other things you might do individually and together to adjust to and appreciate your changing shape?

3. Talk to several mothers and/or couples you admire about their pregnancies. Ask them what they did singly and together during the pregnancy and afterward to keep themselves healthy and positive.

Chapter Five: Finding Out

1. How have you made decisions about which tests (ultrasound, amniocentesis, multiple marker, etc.) to have done during this pregnancy? Talk together about these decisions.

2. If you have had an ultrasound or an amniocentesis, talk to each other about that experience. What surprised you most about seeing and hearing your baby? If your partner could not be present, help him to understand what it was like.

3. If you have learned the gender of your child, how has that affected the way you feel about this pregnancy? If you feel disappointed at first, that's okay. That's a good reason for knowing now, so you can adjust and be ready for your son or daughter. There are always advantages to either gender: your daughter gets a brother; your mom gets a granddaughter; your husband gets a son... There *is* good in this. Often you will discover the benefits later, if not now.

4. If you have learned of a potential health problem, talk about your reaction to that news. Parents who have a

baby with health problems grieve the loss of the healthy baby they expected. They may also have times of resenting the coming baby because of the depth of that child's needs. Since your child is unexpected, your grief and resentment may be even greater than most. Be aware of this and find someone who will let you express your emotions in all their intensity when you need to.

Chapter Six: Starting Over

1. This chapter talks about a life graph and your plans for the future. Where were you as a couple in your life graph before you found out you were pregnant?

2. If you have other children, what part of starting over feels the hardest to you? Is there something you feel you missed out on with your other child/children that perhaps this time you could do differently and better (e.g., nurse longer, work less, divide responsibilities differently, hire more or less childcare, go on dates more often)?

3. Our culture defines success mostly in terms of money, power, and independence. What other measures of success do you think are more important?

4. Are you as successful in these ways right now as you want to be? How could you be more successful together as you move through this pregnancy toward birthing and raising a child?

Chapter Seven: Carrying On

1. You've read about other couples' challenges through their pregnancies. What challenges have you had to face so far, individually and as a couple?

2. We often think we live through our trials alone, that no one sees us. In fact, it is likely that others see you and admire you for continuing with this pregnancy and your life together. What are some of the qualities about you as a couple and as individuals that people would notice and admire?

3. What resources and strategies have you relied on to get you this far?

4. What other resources and strategies do you need now as you approach birth? Make a list of all that you feel you need in terms of supplies (diapers, baby clothes) and emotional support. If you don't have a plan for labor and birth yet, check the books and resources listed at the back of this book to help you prepare.

5. Talk to each other about your anxieties, your excitement, and your concerns regarding labor and birth.

Chapter Eight: Making Changes

1. Making changes in life and in marriage is never easy. It can feel harder when you're in a stressful pregnancy. Yet the pregnancy can help you make decisions and act on them quickly. A deadline is coming soon, and a new life depends on your choices. In a few

sentences, describe to each other the kind of parent
you want to be to your coming son or daughter. Try
writing it down to help clarify, and then preserve
these goals.

2. What kind of changes in your life and in your marriage
do you sense you might need to make to be that kind
of parent? Make a list if that is helpful.

3. Which changes can you make on your own, and
which do you need your partner's help with? Describe
to your partner how he or she could provide the support you need to make these changes.

4. Is there someone in your life—a counselor, pastor,
pregnancy-center volunteer—who you would both
feel comfortable talking to about these changes?

Chapter Nine: Birth

1. If you have already had your baby, congratulations! If
your partner was able to be there with you, talk to
each other about the experience using these questions.

   a. What were you unprepared for? How was it different than you expected?

   b. What surprised and amazed you about your partner during the labor and birth?

   c. If you held your baby in your arms, did you feel
   love for him or her right away, as Pam did, or did
   you feel more like Lori and Jill? Explain.

2. If your partner was not able to be with you, you may be deeply disappointed. You may want to blame him for his absence. Nothing can replace the experience of seeing a child enter the world, but his son or daughter is here now. Try to help him understand what the birth experience was like, then concentrate on moving forward with your child and each other. How does it feel for the three of you to be together right now?

3. If you have chosen to keep this baby, your new life as the parents of this child has just begun. What do you want to do differently in this new life than you've done before? Write down your intentions and desires on a special piece of paper to keep as a reminder of who you want to be as you begin to raise this child.

4. If you haven't had your baby yet, talk to each other about your concerns regarding the coming birth. What words would you choose to describe your feelings as you wait—anxious, excited, elated, exhausted, worried, impatient, apathetic, tense, calm...?

5. Talk to one or more couples you admire who went through birth together. Ask about their birth experiences. Share your concerns with them.

Further Resources

CRISIS PREGNANCY RESOURCES

Web Sites

www.heartbeatinternational.org—Offers quick access to worldwide directory listing 4,883 pregnancy help centers. Most centers provide free pregnancy testing and counseling on abortion alternatives, maternal health, and other needs related to your unexpected pregnancy. This site also contains a search for medical clinics, maternity homes, and nonprofit adoption agencies.

www.nurturingnetwork.org—At this site 42,000 volunteers in 50 states and 25 countries will help you find a positive alternative to abortion. Services include medical assistance, financial assistance, nurturing homes, educational programs,

employment and adoption counseling, and prepa-
ration for parenthood. More than 17,000 mothers
and children served. 1-800-TNN-4MOM

www.pregnancycenters.org—Trained phone consul-
tants are available at all hours to take your calls.
Search can locate the pregnancy center nearest
you, with a map, address, and phone number
provided. 1-800-395-HELP

www.crisispregnancy.com—Complete, one-stop site
providing information on many topics related to
unplanned pregnancy, including teen mothers,
expectant fathers, week-by-week pregnancy calendar, legal considerations, maternity homes, open
adoptions, financial assistance, and more.

www.christiananswers.net/life/home.html—Excellent
source for factual and thoughtful answers on all
aspects of pregnancy, fetal development, and abortion. Deals with such questions as these: When
does life begin? If God knows I'm hurting, why
doesn't he help me? Is abortion justified if a child
is unwanted? Doesn't a woman have the right to
control her own body?

Books

Alban Gosline, Andrea. *Celebrating Motherhood: A
Comforting Companion for Every Expecting Mother.*
Boston: Conari Press, 2002.

Nilsson, Lennart. *A Child Is Born,* 4th ed. New York: Delacorte Press, 2003.

Tsiaras, Alexander. *From Conception to Birth: A Life Unfolds.* New York: Doubleday, 2002.

TEEN PREGNANCY RESOURCES

Web Sites

www.crisispregnancy.com—See the Teen Pregnancy link. Many resources and articles are presented.

www.pregnancy-info.net—See the Teen Pregnancy link. You'll find full access to resources and information.

Books

Davis, Deborah, ed. *You Look Too Young to Be a Mom: Teen Mothers Speak Out on Love, Learning, and Success.* New York: Perigee, 2004.

Goyer, Tricia. *Life Interrupted: The Scoop on Being a Young Mom.* Grand Rapids, MI: Zondervan, 2004.

Perry, Linda Ellen. *How to Survive Your Teen's Pregnancy: Practical Advice for a Christian Family.* Dumfries, VA: Chalfont House, 2003.

Schooler, Jayne E. *Mom, Dad—I'm Pregnant: When Your Daughter or Son Faces an Unplanned Pregnancy.* Colorado Springs: NavPress, 2004.

Williams-Wheeler, Dorrie. *The Unplanned Pregnancy Book for Teens and College Students.* Virginia Beach, VA: Sparkledoll Productions, 2004.

ADOPTION RESOURCES

Web Sites

www.adoption.com—A comprehensive site offering information on all aspects of adoption.

www.bethany.org—An adoption agency. Also offers information and discussion forums. Help line: 1-800-bethany

www.adoptionsbygladney.com—Offers a full range of adoption services, including a residential campus with free housing and assistance throughout the pregnancy and adoption process. 1-817-922-6070 or 1-800-gladney

Books

Dormon, Sara, and Ruth Graham. *I'm Pregnant—Now What? Heartfelt Advice on Getting Through Unplanned Pregnancy.* Ventura, CA: Regal Books, 2004. (focus on teens and adoption)

Lindsay, Jeanne Warren. *Pregnant? Adoption Is an Option.* Buena Park, CA: Morning Glory Press, 1996.

Melina, Lois Ruskai, and Sharon Kaplan Roszia. *The Open Adoption Experience: A Complete Guide for Adoptive and Birth Families—From Making the Decision Through the Child's Growing Years.* New York: HarperPerennial, 1993.

Organizations

Adoptive Families of America

33 Hwy. N

Minneapolis, MN 55422

1-800-372-3300

NEW MOTHER RESOURCES

Web Sites

www.laleche.org—Supports mothers in all aspects of breast-feeding.

www.mops.org—Mothers of Preschoolers offers support groups that meet around the country and resources for mothers of young children.

www.mothersandmore.org—A nonprofit organization dedicated to improving the lives of mothers through support, education, and advocacy. Addresses women's needs as individuals and members of society and promotes the value of all the work mothers do.

www.momsclub.org—Offers support groups, news-
letters, and other resources for mothers at home
with their children. Children are welcome at
meetings.

www.focusonyourchild.com—Full range of comple-
mentary services and resources for parenting
children of every age.

Books

Ketterman, Grace H. *Mothering: An Expert's Guide to
Succeeding in Your Most Important Role.* Nashville:
Nelson, 2001.

Rosenberg, Debra Gilbert, and Mary Sue Miller. *The
New Mom's Companion: Care for Yourself While
You Care for Your Newborn.* Naperville, IL:
Sourcebooks, 2003.

Notes

1. Sarah S. Brown and Leon Eisenberg, eds., *The Best Intentions: Unintended Pregnancy and the Well-Being of Children and Families* (Washington DC: National Academy Press, 1995), 1. "Unintended" is further defined as "mistimed or unwanted" (p. 11). More recent studies cite similar statistics. The American Pregnancy Association cites three million unplanned pregnancies annually. The Population Council, in a report issued September 2000, stated, "Almost as many unintended as intended pregnancies [worldwide] occur each year, and more than half of these unintended pregnancies end in abortion." www.popcouncil.org/publications/popbriefs/pb6(3)_2.html.

2. Voy Forums, www.voy.com, message posted on July 1, 2002.

3. Voy Forums, www.voy.com, message posted on July 27, 2002.

4. Voy Forums, www.voy.com, message posted on November 16, 2004.

5. Sarah S. Brown and Leon Eisenberg, eds., *The Best Intentions: Unintended Pregnancy and the Well-Being of*

Children and Families (Washington DC: National
Academy Press, 1995), 68–72.

6. Anrenée Englander and Corinne Morgan Wilks, ed.,
*Dear Diary, I'm Pregnant: Teenagers Talk About Their
Pregnancy* (Toronto: Annick Press, 1997), 140.

About the Author

Leslie Leyland Fields is the mother of a daughter and five sons, ages seventeen to three. She teaches creative writing in Seattle Pacific University's Master of Fine Arts program and at the University of Alaska. Summers, she works with her family in commercial fishing on a remote island in Alaska. Her essays and poems have been published widely in periodicals such as *The Atlantic, Orion, Christian Science Monitor, Image,* and numerous anthologies. Her books are *Surviving the Island of Grace, Out on the Deep Blue, The Entangling Net,* and *The Water Under Fish.* When not teaching, fishing, or mothering, she speaks at conferences and presents seminars on matters of faith, wilderness, literature, and family. She lives in Kodiak, Alaska, with her husband, Duncan, an ocean resources consultant, and their athletic children, who plan to keep them both on the run (and hopefully young) for many years to come.

For more resources, readers' guides, and other materials related to unexpected pregnancy, see www.surprisechild.com.

Excerpts and photos from Leslie's other books are available at www.leslie-leyland-fields.com.